Managing residential care

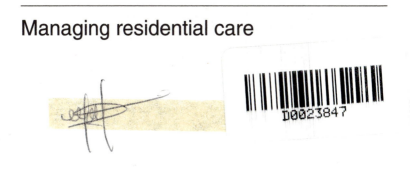

Residential, nursing and children's Homes, and Homes for people with disabilities or with drug, alcohol or mental health problems do not have to be bad places to live; they can be – and occasionally are – the very best places for their residents to thrive. There have been many occasions in the last thirty years when residential care has seemed to be on the brink of a breakthrough – when we could have converted the service into something of which to be universally proud.

Managing Residential Care analyses what is wrong and proposes how residential care can be managed well. It covers the economic and political contexts of residential care, the practicalities of managing care, and the roles of outside organisations, including inspection, local authorities, charities, private care companies and housing associations. Extended examples throughout the text demonstrate both how managers can succeed and how the powerful forces of mismanagement obstruct them.

Managing Residential Care will be essential reading for residential care practitioners and managers, training officers and policy makers, and lecturers and students on social work and social care courses.

John Burton is an Independent Social Care Consultant. He has also written *The Handbook of Residential Care*.

Managing residential care

John Burton

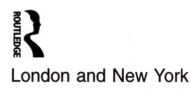

London and New York

First published 1998 by Routledge
11 New Fetter Lane, London EC4P 4EE

Simultaneously published in the USA and Canada
by Routledge
29 West 35th Street, New York, NY 10001

© 1998 John Burton

Typeset in Times by Keystroke, Jacaranda Lodge, Wolverhampton
Printed and bound in Great Britain by Creative Print and Design
(Wales), Ebbw Vale

British Library Cataloguing in Publication Data
A catalogue record for this book is available from the British Library

Library of Congress Cataloging in Publication Data
Burton, John, 1947–
    Managing residential care / John Burton.
        p.   cm.
    Includes bibliographical references and index.
    1. Institutional care—Great Britain—Management. I. Title.
    HV63.G7B88 1998
    361′.05—dc21   97–18305
                                                CIP

ISBN 0–415–16487–7 (hbk)
ISBN 0–415–16488–5 (pbk)

Contents

Preface

I was woken several times last night by the raucous, demented ranting
of a neighbour. She stands at her open window shouting to the street.
Sometimes I can make out the words but mostly she shouts them so fast
and furiously, interspersing them with growls and yelps, that I can hear
only the sound of her pain and distress. This woman is in mental agony;
she needs help.

She lives in a block of flats which is part of 'care in the community'.
She should be being cared for in a residential Home or she may even
need to be in hospital at the moment, but it is too expensive to care
for her properly and, in any case, there are no places available, so, like
hundreds of other people in this area, she has been discarded into the
'community'.

This part of Brixton, in South London, is indeed a caring community,
but the implementation of community care has not made it any more
caring and may have made it less. I have lived in this street for twenty-
seven years – more than half my life. Many of my neighbours have lived
here longer. It is one of the most economically deprived wards in the
whole country. Unemployment, especially amongst young Black men,
is very high. Brixton was the first part of Britain in which Caribbean
people made their homes in the late 1940s and the 1950s. Several of my
neighbours, now retired or near retirement, were among the founders
and builders of the Welfare State. Since then people from all over
the world and of all cultures and religions have come to live in this
community. Neighbours know and help each other, but the young Black
woman in the 'community care' flats needs more than can be offered
by neighbours, however caring. Perhaps a desperate community care
manager thought Brixton was a suitable place for her, but no one knows
her and she doesn't know the neighbourhood. She has been dumped.
Other people who live in the flats are a part of the community, yet,

because of the 'community care' policies of the council and the health authority, they are being moved. The small local charity which used to support the residents of the flats has been closed down; its bid for the contract was unsuccessful. A big housing association has taken over.

In another part of Brixton, an old people's Home stands boarded up and empty, windows broken, garden overgrown. Outside a notice proclaims that it will be auctioned. For many years the council invested hundreds of thousands of pounds in this building. Staff made heroic efforts to improve the service to the residents and, until it was closed two years ago, they were succeeding. The remaining residents were 'resettled' elsewhere – to other homes which are now also being closed. Those who didn't die in the first move will probably die this time round. Throughout the last thirty years of its existence the Home was mis-managed but everything that went wrong was blamed on the staff.

In an adjacent borough, private care companies flourish by employing too few staff and paying them a pittance. The inspection unit is in the pocket of the politicians and senior managers, and there is no one to protect residents from exploitation and abuse. In the same borough a voluntary organisation providing services for people with drug problems pays its residential workers less than its day-care workers. The care staff in another voluntary organisation run by powerful and wealthy local politicians earn barely £3 an hour. To supplement their wages, they are allowed to take home food, cleaning materials and lavatory paper.

Here in Brixton, the local authority has given up running its own children's Homes. It now sends children far away to privately run Homes or to foster homes set up by private fostering agencies. Often the social workers know little about the placements, but the managers console themselves by remembering how their own Homes were just as bad but even more expensive.

Most of the social care jobs advertised in the *Guardian* and *Community Care* each week are for relatively highly paid managers who will only rarely have contact with anyone who uses their service. Many of those who actually do the caring – short-term, part-time, temporary, poorly paid workers – are recruited by the staff agencies.

I began writing this book at a time when this dispiriting outlook threatened my own strong beliefs in the positive potential of residential care. The job of a manager committed to providing good residential care was to struggle on, holding tightly to values and principles, in the hope that some day the tide would turn. I finish writing soon after the general election of 1997. I now have a firmer grasp on my optimism. After eighteen years of a government hostile to the idea that we have communal responsibilities for looking after each other, we now have a government whose leader accepts that we do share responsibility for each other's welfare. It remains to be seen whether this different thinking leads to truly different practice. I very much hope it does. We – you and I – have a part to play in the outcome.

My first experience of residential care was in 1965 and I was optimistic then. I have been involved with the work ever since. I have written on the basis of my long and varied – and mostly good – experience of being a residential care worker and manager, an inspector, a consultant, a management committee member and a teacher of residential work. I have worked with hundreds of people who actually do the job well and with just a few managers who manage it well. Good residential workers manage most of their work themselves, and a central theme of the book is that residential care in fact is better managed within the Home, rather than by outsiders.

There is very little in this book about independent consultancy – the work I do now – helping staff teams and managers to develop better residential services. Yet, of course, writing and reading this book is in itself a consultative act. As I have written, I have constantly imagined myself to be in conversation with you; so when I write 'we' in the book, I do not mean some pompous 'royal we', I mean a 'you and me' we. I hope that as a reader you will gain awareness and insight, reflect on your practice, take a helpfully critical view of your organisation, and understand more how the 'system' works and how it might be changed to work better. You may also use the practical advice which I offer. But, above all, I hope that reading the book helps you to strengthen your resolve, and to find your own ways of managing good residential care, creating good places for people to live their lives – or a period of their lives – in and to get the support they need.

John Burton, May 1997
42 Hetherington Road, Brixton, London SW4 7PA
0171-733 5230

Acknowledgements

Hundreds of people have contributed to this book over many years. I have learned from excellent practitioners and managers – and from some very poor ones! Some readers may think that they momentarily recognise themselves or the other people, places and incidents I write about; however, although based on my real experience, all the stories I tell and the examples I set out are made up. None of the characters in them is a real, identifiable person. I am grateful to all the people I have worked with over so many years, and say to them, 'If the character is unflattering, it isn't you! But if you think I've borrowed a bit of your brilliance to create this individual, take the credit.' (If that doesn't get you to read the book, nothing will.)

It's dangerous to mention anyone by name because each time I think of one person, I immediately think of a dozen others whom I should thank. However, residential care *is* risky, so to demonstrate my daring, and in the sincere hope that mentioning any of you here will not ruin the rest of your career (if you still have one), I want to thank the following: Eileen Donohoe and Ina Burford for their inspiration; Sylvia Ballard for her affection, and her indomitable character and spirit; Chris Beedell, Bruce Senior and Des Sowerby for their wisdom and friendship; Josie Jennings for her courage in standing up for what was right; Aileen Alleyne for combining friendship with illuminating professional talk; David Gurman for keeping me in touch and boosting my spirits; Mike Stephenson and Sheila Macdonald for their affirmation and for being good to work with; two important Barbaras – Kahan and Dockar-Drysdale – and Isobel Menzies (none of whom I know) for the enormous amount I have gained from their writing; Shadikul Haque for calling round and being a friend; Phyl Burton for her aesthetic, creative and practical management; Val Rowlands for her knowledge and tenacity, and her hatred of injustice; Elizabeth Burton for nearly everything else(!) but especially for talking over many of the issues in this book and so often providing unusual insights; and Tim Burton for again helping me throughout with the craft and sheer hard work of writing.

And, of course, I thank all you others who have just thrown the book down in disgust: 'To think of all I did for him, the ungrateful ***!'

Introduction

The purpose of this book is to promote the development of residential care through better management. Residential Homes are bedevilled by poor management at all levels. No amount of good intentions on the part of the managing organisation will translate into good care unless the Home itself is well managed from the inside. However, it is rare for the manager of a Home (the care manager) to be sufficiently determined (and lucky) to resist the management failures of the organisation which runs the Home. Therefore, for good residential care to become an established reality, both 'inside' and 'outside' management must work together towards one goal – meeting residents' needs. This book is written for everyone involved: managers, care workers, residents and their relatives, advocates, inspectors, local and national politicians, directors of organisations which provide care, management committee members, policy-makers, students, and social care educators and trainers.

There are four main parts. Part I (Chapters 1–5) comprises five 'stories' of management ranging from the care worker in a small Home who, while she is the one person on duty, is also the person in charge and therefore 'manages', to the director of care services for a large housing association. A wide range of Homes and managers are described, and these stories and characters are used and further developed as examples in subsequent chapters. All the people and places are listed at the beginning of Part I.

In Part II (Chapters 6 and 7) the reader is invited to think about residential care: its status and purpose, its past and present context, and the ways in which it is managed and organised now. Chapter 7 introduces the idea of residential care as a 'therapeutic social ecology'.

Part III (Chapters 8–12) attends to the practicalities of managing residential care, beginning with responding to residents' needs, and power and participation (Chapter 8). Staffing Homes and managing the workforce are discussed in detail in Chapter 9. The physical environment and the financial management of Homes are the subjects of Chapters 10 and 11. The final chapter in Part III – 'Putting it all together and making it work: the therapeutic ecology in action' – demonstrates how all the complex practical aspects of managing residential care must be brought together in an integrated whole in order to provide a good service for residents.

In Part IV (Chapters 13–15) we again look outside the Home to the political and economic environment of residential care – to those outsiders who have so much influence and must take so much of the responsibility for the current state of the service. We propose that 'inside/outside' roles, relationships and responsibilities must be radically reformed, because in general outside power is currently misused, inappropriate and obstructive. In each of the three chapters in this part we examine, in turn, the organisations which manage residential Homes, the 'policy élite' and the independent outsiders – notably inspectors.

Finally, in the Afterword, we set out proposals for change based on the analysis provided in the book.

The following words and phrases are used in particular ways:

- *Home* with a capital H means a residential care or nursing Home.
- *Care manager*, care/nursing team manager, unit manager, Home manager and head of Home are all used to describe the 'inside' manager of a Home. Care manager is also commonly used as the title for the social services worker who assesses clients in the 'community' and 'purchases' services on their behalf.
- The *primary task* is the central purpose of the organisation (or Home), the proper focus of its work – the job without which it has no legitimate reason for functioning.
- *Black/White* is not used as a description of someone's 'race'. ('Race' is itself not a scientific but a political description.) In circumstances in which people's colour and ethnic heritage influence their own and other people's attitudes and actions – favourably or unfavourably – the words Black and White are used as a 'political' description of where the people stand in relation to those attitudes and actions (e.g. racism). Black/White is clearly not an accurate description of colour

and the term is therefore given a capital letter to denote that it is used in a similar way to Asian, European, African, etc. As attitudes, cultures and politics change, so do words and their usage.

Part I

Five stories of management

People and places

Chapter 1 The Una Marson Project
A small residential Home for women who have been dependent on illegal drugs. (The Home is named after Una Marson (1905–65) a Jamaican feminist writer and social worker, who lived and worked in England in the 1930s and 1940s.)

Marcia - care worker
Sally - care worker

Chapter 2 The Drive
A local authority children's Home.

Bob - new manager
Clive - retired manager of another Home in the same local authority
Sonya - Bob's predecessor at The Drive
Kylie - resident
Ellen - domestic care worker
Paul (Chapter 6) - resident at The Drive during the time when Sonya was manager

Chapter 3 The Limes
A private Home for adults with learning disabilities.

Noreen - manager/co-proprietor
Reg - Noreen's husband and co-proprietor
Thomas - new manager
Ann (Chapter 8) - resident
Brenda (Chapter 15) - Noreen's sister, who works in a Home in another area

Chapter 4 The residential and day care section of a local authority social services department

Norwood House - a large 'resource centre' for older people
Lok - service manager
Rachel - manager of Norwood House
Mr Brown (Chapter 8) - resident of Norwood House

Chapter 5 The care services division of Hetherington Housing Trust

Janet - Director of Care Services
Jeeva - Care Services Manager
Hyacinth (Chapter 12) - senior care worker in a nursing Home
Mr Scott (Chapter 12) - resident in the same nursing Home

Chapter 1

Marcia

Marcia is one of five full-time care workers at the Una Marson Project. She has arrived at midday on Saturday at the beginning of her weekend shift. She is taking over from Sally who started at midday on Friday and will leave as soon as she has given the 'handover' to Marcia.

The Una Marson Project is a residential Home for up to seven women who are trying to end their dependency on illegal drugs and/or alcohol. In practice, all the women who come to this Home have used illegal drugs, and although some are also drinkers, they are all here to attempt to free themselves from the addictive illegal drug culture in which they have become enmeshed. Most of them genuinely intend to make a go of it – even those (perhaps especially those) for whom the stark alternative to residence at the Una Marson Project was a prison sentence. There is room for residents' children at Una Marson and there are three young children in the house on this Saturday.

Marcia is not surprised when she learns that the 'relief' worker who was meant to be working from 11 a.m. to 7 p.m. today has not turned up yet, and is not responding to Sally's phone calls. Sally has left messages for two other relief workers to see if they can come in, but has had no response. The house is supposed to have two members of staff on duty during the busy parts of the day but, due to the unreliability of staff, it frequently has only one.

Marcia has been at the project as a permanent team member for six months now; before that she was a relief worker. She has worked in several residential projects but wanted to come to Una Marson in particular because it was for women only, because children could accompany their mothers, and because a good proportion of the residents and the staff were Black. It was important to her that services for people having problems with drugs were seen to be genuinely multiracial and that didn't mean just having the occasional isolated Black resident, or one Black member of staff in a team of six. In Marcia's experience, which was considerable, most drugs projects were like that, and, in the past, she had frequently felt that she was employed only on the grounds that she was a Black woman, which helped previous employers to show that their equal opportunities policy was working. At Una Marson four of the team, including the project manager, and a little less than half the regular relief workers are Black.

Sally, from whom Marcia was receiving the 'handover', is White. She's been at the project for just over a year and is pretty good in Marcia's view. She is in fact an ex-user who, as a client, had been to several 'de-toxes' and projects like the Una Marson before really being able, after long struggles with repeated failures, to come back into the area as a worker. She brings with her a deep understanding of addiction which makes her a dedicated and reliable colleague who, as far as Marcia knows, has never let the project or a resident down. She's also pretty tough-minded about the work. She is intolerant of sloppiness, which she and Marcia agree is too evident in this and most other similar projects. While she understands many of the residents' problems only too well, she is also clear, reliable and utterly unsentimental with them. Sally likes this work and, for all its faults, the Una Marson is the best place she has worked in so far. She realises that there are strong elements of management in the work she is now doing, but she has no ambition to become a manager. Indeed, she feels that she is quite likely still to be here, doing the same job, in five years' time – and still enjoying it. In this respect Marcia is different. She, too, understands that much of her present work entails management, even though she hasn't yet achieved that title, but – unlike Sally – she does want to become a manager.

Sally and Marcia are both annoyed that the relief worker has not turned up. Marcia suspects that she has gone to the carnival even though she made a firm commitment to come to work. The residents will certainly assume that is the reason for her absence.

After much discussion between staff and residents, both together and separately, and after taking a formal decision in the 'house meeting' on the previous Wednesday, it had been decided that Marcia would go to the carnival with three of the residents and with the 5- and 7-year-old children. The relief worker was not included in any of these discussions, and now, by not coming into work, it looks as if she has prevented the residents from going to the carnival.

Marcia and Sally discuss the situation. Two of the residents have got ready and, dressed in their best clothes, the children who were due to go are playing excitedly in the front room. The residents are aware that the relief worker has not turned up, but appear to be ignoring the implications. They have learned to trust Marcia; when she says she's going to do something she generally does it. However, like Marcia, they do not trust the place – in other words, the team and organisation.

Sally has to go soon. She is taking her 15-year-old son shopping and out for a meal. She has painstakingly rebuilt this relationship over the last five years and she is determined not to let him down. If someone doesn't come in soon, the carnival outing will have to be cancelled. Or, Sally and Marcia are now debating, perhaps the two residents who are still keen could take their children by themselves. It is the family day of the carnival and the main purpose is to go to see the floats, dancers and bands, but the risks for the women are huge. There will be intense pressure to relapse at an event where it is very hard to resist the easy availability of alcohol and drugs. It was risky enough with Marcia present, as originally planned, and this was much discussed at the staff and house meetings. One of the residents has been at the project for only two weeks and readily accepts that she needs the extra control of staff presence for a while yet. It would be courting failure for her to go on her own. As she thinks about the situation, Marcia suddenly becomes quite furious with the relief worker for her irresponsibility and casualness. Her fury distracts her from thinking constructively about what to do and how to manage this situation. Time is getting on. She and Sally have now been talking together in the little office for more than forty minutes and they are still no nearer a solution. The midday meal, which one of the residents has prepared for everyone, is now ready; the plan was for the carnival-goers to leave at 1 p.m. Marcia is momentarily lost in her anger, when one of the residents who is ready for the outing comes to the door and asks, 'When are we going?' Marcia, still full of her fury, turns on the resident and says bitterly, 'It doesn't look as if we are going.' The resident, who is quick to accept bad news and make it worse, does not stop to discuss it, but storms out of the room shouting, 'I knew we wouldn't go. You can't trust anyone in this fucking place.' She goes into the front room and shouts at her children, 'Get changed back into your play clothes. We're not going to the carnival.'

Sally, now fearful that she cannot leave Marcia on her own with this developing situation and that she may be compelled to let her son down, picks up the phone in one last attempt to get assistance. She phones the manager, who doesn't usually work at weekends but always says she can be telephoned in an emergency. To Sally's relief, the manager is in. She is just about to set off to the carnival with her own young children.

She says that she will call round to the project on her way and any residents who want to go, can go with her.

Marcia's grateful to Sally for making that arrangement, but is left with a jumble of feelings and thoughts about what has happened. To her it is ironic that with such seeming ease the manager is going to solve what had become an impossible situation. In addition to her intense annoyance with the individual relief worker, Marcia feels that it is continuing poor management throughout this project, and so many others like it, which has led to this situation, and which repeatedly lets down residents who should be able to trust the place. And now the manager will swan in and solve the problem as if it had never happened. All the planning with residents and the encouragement to them to take control and responsibility is shown to be wasted time and effort. Yet again, they have experienced that they are wholly at the mercy of events, of whims and chance; and so, they may well ask, what's the point of trying to take charge of your life?

But Marcia is still left with the whole situation in the house to manage for the rest of the day, the evening, the night and Sunday morning. Marcia and Sally go to the kitchen, where some residents are already sitting, starting their lunch. Marcia, unenthusiastically, summarises the revised plan to the residents, and Sally says goodbye, hopes they have a good afternoon and tells them she will see them again on Monday.

One of the residents who had said at the house meeting that she wanted to go to the carnival had already had a bad morning. (This formed part of the report which Sally had given Marcia in the first part of their handover meeting.) She has been lying on her bed in her room for much of the morning, refusing to talk about her fear of being exposed to the temptations and threats of the outing. Just before lunch, one of the other residents came up to tell her that the outing was off, so she came down to lunch confident that she could behave as if it was not her decision and that she would have gone if only the staff could have got themselves together. She is rather nonplussed by Marcia's announcement that the outing is now going to take place after all.

There are several more hiccups before the group finally leaves for the carnival with the manager and her two small children. She had turned up later than they thought she might and the children at the project had become fractious and one had torn her new dress. There had been arguments and the reluctant resident had used the lateness of the manager and the impatient atmosphere to extricate herself once more and retire to the safety of her room. When the manager did eventually arrive, she was in her car, which, though large, was not really suitable to take two more adults, three children and her own two children. Nevertheless, they did all squeeze in, but only two of the children in the back seat were properly secured with suitable safety belts. Originally, it had been planned that Marcia would take the group on the bus. She was looking forward to taking them, not only because she would have liked to have gone to the carnival herself, but mostly because she had thought about it, and planned it, and was going to make it a thoroughly enjoyable and productive outing for the residents and their children.

By the time the group leaves, Marcia is tired and very fed up. She feels she has been implicated in yet another sloppy bit of work. She resolves to retrieve what is left of the day and to make sure that the time is productive for at least some of the five women who are left behind.

The resident who opted out of going to the carnival is still upstairs and Marcia thinks it would be wrong to give her attention under these circumstances, especially since there are four other residents, who often miss out because they are less demanding. It is planned that all the residents have individual time with their key workers during the week – although it doesn't always work out that way. Marcia feels that the weekends and evenings should make use of the group and communal nature of the household – doing things together – although it is always possible for individuals to opt out. It is a warm, sunny day. On several weekends in the last month, Marcia has got residents involved in the garden at the back of the house outside the kitchen. It's looking pretty now, but the lawn needs cutting and there are a lot of other little jobs to do. The four other residents are sitting watching an old film on TV.

First Marcia gets out the gardening tools. She bought them (with project money) and collected some others together in the spring, shortly after she started in her permanent post, and she keeps them tidily and securely. Even if she doesn't use them every time she's on duty, she usually checks that they are there, and her colleagues have learned that the surest way to upset Marcia is to leave one of the tools lying around or the lawn mower out. Rather ostentatiously she puts the shears, trowel, fork, secateurs and broom outside the sitting room window in full view of the couch potatoes inside. She then starts cutting the grass but stops after a few minutes.

Marcia goes inside. She checks the contents of the fridge and gets herself a glass of water with a lot of ice in it. She takes this with her into the sitting room and asks the resident who is responsible for preparing the evening meal what she's cooking. 'Chicken,' she answers

– without interest and affecting annoyance at being interrupted from watching the film. 'Mm, you don't fancy a barbecue, do you?' says Marcia, who knows perfectly well what's for supper and is pretty sure, by that time, that they are all going to have a delightful barbecue when the carnival-goers come back at about 7.30 p.m.

Without waiting for an answer to her proposal, Marcia returns to the garden and resumes her energetic lawn mowing. Within a few minutes, one by one, the four telly-watchers emerge into the sunlight and in no time they are beginning to join in. One takes over the mower, another starts to snip dead heads off roses, and another sweeps the paving. Marcia goes with the cook to find some herbs and spices in which to marinate the chicken. Later the hose is brought out and after a bit of serious watering, all five women, including Marcia, get into a ridiculous game, charging around, screaming and squirting each other with the hose.

The resident upstairs is woken by the screams, looks out of her window, and staggers down to join in the fun.

They all sit around in the sun sipping iced fruit juice and listening to tapes, and then still together, they start to prepare the meal, putting a table and chairs outside, setting up the barbecue, and making salads and desserts, each of them having some special idea to contribute.

By the time the carnival-goers return at about 7.45, the chicken is nearly cooked and the meal is set out enticingly on the table. Everyone is in a good mood, except for those who went on the outing. They return tired and arguing amongst themselves. The manager had more or less 'dropped them off', just stopping for a couple of minutes to tell Marcia that the outing was 'fine' in spite of a couple of mishaps which the residents would tell her about. One of the residents insisted that she should see the table set out and almost dragged her through to the garden. Marcia tried to persuade her to stay for a while and have a drink and something to eat with everyone, but the manager explained she had to rush off to prepare a meal at home. Her own children were very reluctant to leave.

In amongst the fun and enjoyment of the afternoon and early evening, Marcia had also been thinking about the return of the outing, and the rest of her shift until tomorrow morning. She made sure that the woman in charge of the barbecue remembered the dangers to three small, tired children. Often the residents without children could be very sensible and caring with the other women's children. Even that depended very much on which worker was on duty and what example they set. Without making an issue out of it, Marcia had spoken with most of the residents about how tired the children (and their mothers) might be when they returned. Her idea was to have the meal virtually ready, so that the children could sit down and enjoy the atmosphere and the food, and tell them all about the carnival. She did not want tired children, full of the exciting (and perhaps disturbing) experiences of the afternoon, racketing around, being shouted at but not attended to by their mothers, grabbing bits of food and drinks, and spoiling their own day and everyone else's. Marcia was therefore very firm about them all sitting down at the table and she sat with them and really concentrated on what they said about the afternoon. Two of the other residents also sat down while the other three started bringing the food and drinks. Marcia established the atmosphere and then held it. The children retold the story of the outing, what they had seen: the noise and music, the people all dressed up, the dancing, the clowns, the drunk man, the witch, the monster . . . and how one of them had got lost and how the others found him. It was heady stuff.

Everything went well. It was unusual to have such a convivial atmosphere at any time in the project. At about 9 p.m. the children were beginning to droop; the 5-year-old was fast asleep, sitting on her mother's lap. When they got up to take the children to bed, Marcia said to both mothers, 'Stay with them till they're asleep.'

The rest of the group stayed up, sitting talking around the table. This meal had reminded them of many good things and also of people, places and relationships they had lost. The woman who had successfully avoided the carnival trip, talked a lot and for the first time felt she was part of the group.

Later, while the residents started to clear up, Marcia took the log-book and notes into the sitting room. She tried to record individual and group events fully and accurately. What she omitted were some of her own thoughts and feelings which she came face to face with as she reflected on the day. While she recorded the fact that the relief worker had not turned up, she did not write of her fury; while the fortunate intervention of the manager was acknowledged, the lack of planning, and the many other aspects of poor management which the outing had epitomised to Marcia, were not mentioned. Nor did Marcia include her realisation that at least some of her energy and motivation for managing such an excellent afternoon and evening came from her anger and her determination to demonstrate that she could make this place work through a combination of precise planning, sharp awareness and creativity. Marcia had not stopped working since she came in through the door at midday. It was now 11 p.m. The perfect way to round off this day would be to get to bed before midnight, to have a good night's sleep (unusual when 'sleeping in'), and to be fit to work the next day.

Marcia was still writing the notes when three of the residents who had been clearing up came into the sitting room. One switched on the telly and the other two slumped down on the sofa. Marcia is first horrified – then annoyed with the residents – and then with herself for forgetting that the residents nearly always watch the late film on a Saturday night, especially if it's a horror film. Nevertheless, she says, 'Oh no, you're not going to watch telly are you? . . . I can't bear it. I thought I was going to get to bed early.' The residents don't really take much notice of her protestations, because this late night is an agreement, made in the house meeting, and the residents know that Marcia sticks to agreements. Wearily, Marcia gets up and says, 'I'm making some tea; who wants a cup?'

When she returns with the tea, one of the residents tells her to write in the notes that today was one of the best days she'd ever had in her whole life. Marcia believes her, and she knows that, in spite of all the obstacles, it was she who managed it that way.

Chapter 2

Bob

Bob is the recently appointed manager of 24 The Drive, a local authority Home for children and young people. He has now been in the job for nearly a month. He was previously a senior worker in another Home in the same authority. He completed his Diploma in Social Work (DipSW) about a year ago after working in residential child care for the past ten years.

This job seemed to be the logical step forward. He has worked his way up in this authority, having started as a temporary worker after university and then working in various Homes in the voluntary and local authority sectors, sometimes as a permanent member of staff and sometimes working through an agency. Before he did his Diploma in Social Work, he had been the acting head of another Home, after the previous officer in charge had retired on medical grounds. Although the Home had very few residents and only four permanent staff, this had been useful experience for Bob to add to his CV. Nothing had gone seriously wrong during his time in charge of the Home – which had closed soon after he went on his diploma course – and the local authority was grateful to him for standing in as 'caretaker' for six months.

That Home had quite a history, and both the previous officer in charge, Clive, and the local authority were pleased to have 'let go' of the place with so little fuss. Most people in the 'children and families' division of the social services department were aware of long-standing rumours and doubts about the Home, though it had been a useful resource to the department for many years, with a reputation for coping with some very difficult teenagers. Some social workers who were 'well in' with Clive contrived to get places for their clients even when the official line was that the Home was full. He tended to run things the way he wanted them, and he was admired for being so down-to-earth and independent, and for not caring much what his managers thought or said. They had never done the job, and in his view knew nothing about it. As far as he was concerned, you either 'had it' or you didn't. Some adolescents appeared to flourish there, but others either complained and left, or were slung out. Most social workers who had to place children considered it worth cultivating Clive and ignoring his 'odd' behaviour and attitudes. For some years he and the previous director of social services had been drinking friends, and he was on similar terms with two influential councillors. When a new director was appointed, she was made aware of some of the complaints, and instigated an initial investigation. Clive almost immediately went sick and after ten months was retired on grounds of ill health. Bob was then put in charge for the last six months before the Home was closed. It is rumoured that Clive is now in a business partnership with the previous director of social services in another part of the country, and they are setting up a company to run private children's homes, a service to escort children and young people to and from court, and a social care consultancy.

Bob has never been employed in any capacity in a Home which really works. He certainly has plenty of experience in years, but it is poor experience. While he was on his DipSW course, he selected placements in field work teams, partly because of his extensive residential work experience and partly because he wanted to transfer to field work after qualifying. He had not used the training course to reflect on, investigate and refine his residential care knowledge and experience – indeed, he avoided the subject and rather despised it – but the officer in charge post came up at 24 The Drive and he was tempted by being able to earn at least 50 per cent more than he would have received as a newly qualified social worker. He hadn't spent ten years on a sub-standard salary in residential work only to take a drop now that he was qualified.

The first month at The Drive had been hard. Sonya, the previous manager, had built up a good reputation, so good that the central managers had decided that she should move to take over a slightly larger Home which had long-standing problems. She was seen to be the solution to such problems. The staff team at the Drive, which had a core of good workers, was resentful about the loss of their respected manager and, as it seemed to them, the imposition of a new manager who appeared to share few of their ideals and aspirations for the Home. He was also associated with the closure of the Home at which he had been the temporary manager more than two years before. The staff team were convinced that Bob's appointment meant that The Drive would be the next Home to close. The residents, too, most of whom had lived at the Home while the previous manager had been there, resented Bob's intrusion. More ready than the staff to voice the thoughts and feelings they were nursing, the young people openly rejected his criticisms of the Home and opposed his proposals for change. Within a couple of weeks, Bob was regretting his mercenary motives for taking the job. 'It's just not worth the hassle,' he would mutter to himself several times a day.

His way of coping with the situation was to attempt to detach himself. He resolved to work 'office hours' from Monday to Friday. (This move was approved of by the headquarters managers and had been recommended by the local inspection unit. Both said they wanted to see more 'professional' management in residential Homes, and were sure that such working hours were a true sign of professionalism.) Bob had taken to wearing a suit or a jacket and tie, and carrying a briefcase. He went to all the meetings at head office and spent much of his time when he was actually in the Home sitting at the computer writing the documents – policies and procedures – which the inspectors, at more than one inspection, had reported were absent. Weekly staff meetings had become well established in the Home under the previous regime and all staff were rostered to be on duty on the day of the meeting. Bob found the first two meetings painfully negative and was worried about his staffing budget. He announced that in future there would be a meeting once a fortnight. Any staff who were off duty but wished to attend would be able to take an hour and a half off as soon as the opportunity presented itself. Bob had never worked in a Home where staff meetings were any more than protracted grumbles or, alternatively, a time for the manager to say what he or she wanted and ask if anyone had any questions at the end. So he couldn't understand the passionate attachment which the team at The Drive showed to their staff meetings, and he had no idea of the depth of insult which they felt when he said he thought they were a waste of time and money.

Today, Monday, Bob arrives at The Drive as usual at 9 a.m. He parks his new car (which came with the job) at the front of the large 1970s building and lets himself in. He has a lot to do today. He has to complete the writing of the Home's policy on sanctions and the admissions procedure, and, having been in post for a whole month, he wants to bring all his financial figures up to date so that he can check on spending and the projections for the rest of the year. He will take these figures to the staff meeting on Wednesday, so that all staff can be well aware of the financial constraints within which they have to work. On the staffing costs, by far the major part of the budget, he has worked out exactly how much the staff meeting was costing and is able to show that the new arrangements will release sufficient funds to allow an additional member of staff to be on duty most weekends. However, for the moment, he will argue, there is a massive projected overspend, so they will have to find savings wherever possible. There will be no overtime; everyone is to take time off in lieu ('TOIL') of any additional hours worked within a week of accruing them, and no agency staff whatsoever will be used until they get the spending under control. The current vacancy in a team of twelve (including him) will not be filled until the new financial year. These are Bob's preoccupations as he unlocks the door to his office and automatically switches on his computer.

Elsewhere in the building some staff and residents have very different concerns. It has been a difficult weekend. One of the residents, Kylie, a thin and immature 15-year-old girl, who was close to the previous officer in charge and whose behaviour has deteriorated ever since she left, has 'trashed' her room. This happened shortly after the return at 2 a.m. on Sunday of two of the boys (aged 15 and 16) from the local police station, where they had been charged with breaking into a shop. They had been caught in the act. The out-of-hours social worker had been called out by the residential workers who were 'sleeping in' to act as 'responsible adult' to them at the police station, because the staff couldn't leave the premises. The boys returned to the Home in a police van, drunk and high on the story of their daring (but very clumsy) break-in. They wanted food and insisted on trying to cook themselves something, and they still had cans of strong lager with them which they refused to hand over to the two staff. They burned the food and in doing so set the fire alarm off, waking those residents who were not already awake. When eventually they did go upstairs, they racketed around, going in and out of their rooms and banging on other children's doors. They knocked repeatedly on Kylie's door until eventually she opened it and then they threw the remains of their cans of lager over her, shouting out, 'It's a wet T-shirt competition'. Kylie, frightened and humiliated, retreated into her room, put a chair under the door handle, and proceeded to wreck everything. She tore up her clothes, smashed her pictures and her stereo, threw the curtains and bedding out of the window, and eventually, exhausted and sobbing, and with a torn sheet wrapped around her, she curled up in a corner and slept.

The two staff on duty, a man and a woman, had done their very best to minimise the danger of the incident. However, they had not known that Kylie had 'trashed' her room until the following morning at 8 a.m. when one of them, staring wearily out of the kitchen window, sipping a mug of coffee, saw the curtains and bedclothes strewn across the garden. She then went upstairs, and slowly and gently coaxed Kylie into opening her door.

Saturday evening had been fairly pleasant and uneventful, partly because the two boys were out of the house. At 11.30 p.m. they had to be 'reported missing' to the police; but when the staff went to bed at about midnight they were hoping that the boys would not be found and would stay out all night. Reporting them missing had become a routine response to their frequent absences; and when they were in the Home they were always in trouble and there was little that the staff could do about it. Although they were known to be up to no good, and their rooms were cluttered with stolen goods, no one felt they had the authority or power to step in and call a halt either to their behaviour or to their continuing stay at the Home. The staff had lost heart. It was thought that sooner or later they would get involved in some crime which would result in custody; only in that way would the home be rid of them and their impossible behaviour.

The staff had tried to discuss the ruinous effect of the boys' presence in the Home at the first two staff meetings which Bob had attended. It sounded to him as if they were simply whining about their jobs. After all, as he pointed out, he hadn't accepted them as residents; they were already in the Home when he took over. Ironically, they had been moved from the troublesome Home to which Sonya, the former head of The Drive, had recently gone as manager. Simply moving young people to another Home was the main way in which the local authority's most difficult children in care were 'worked with'. In his view it was this staff team and Sonya (who was considered to be so good at handling difficult teenagers) who had accepted the boys. It was not up to him now to turn round to his line manager and ask for the boys to be moved; it might appear that he couldn't handle the first difficult residents he was presented with. He told the staff that it was their job to work with all residents. Meanwhile, he said, he would be reviewing the admissions procedure and particularly the Home's policy on sanctions, because, in his view, the staff had been inconsistent in the way they responded to the boys' bad behaviour, and they had got away with far more than they should have done.

As Bob starts work in his office, he is completely unaware of the events of the weekend which are now being discussed in the kitchen by the two child-care workers who have slept in on Sunday night and the domestic worker. They too are seeking solace in detachment – 'It's not our fault' – and they agree together that Sonya would not have let things get to this stage. The domestic worker, Ellen, has worked at the Home since it opened in 1977.

It took a long time for Ellen to accept Sonya's 'therapeutic' ways of working, but once she got involved and was given increasing recognition and responsibility, she began to love her job and to thrive in it. She felt a very full part of the team and made skilful and significant contributions to therapeutic work. She is angry with what Bob is doing in the Home. Suddenly she has become nothing more than a cleaner again. But apart from having a good moan about the situation, and entrenching their dislike of and antagonism to the two bad boys, this discussion does not get Ellen and the two care workers anywhere in terms of managing the situation for all the young people in residence.

Although the staff and some of the young people know that Bob is in because they've seen his car, and in any case he's always in at 9 a.m., no one goes to tell him what has happened during the night. If he had read the log-book as soon as he arrived he would know what has happened; but that is not his habit. He reads the log-book when he goes to get his coffee at 10.30 a.m. each day – and he calls this 'management monitoring'. Of course, he has said that he is to be called if there is ever a 'real emergency'; but the weekend staff judged that the night's events never became what Bob would term a real emergency. Because of his detached attitude, they now gave him little information – and that, grudgingly. They felt he wasn't going to help them and that he avoided difficult situations in the Home, so they weren't going to tell him anything. They also felt that the only reason he would want to be told of problems was that if ever he had to deal with his own line management, he would put the blame on the staff, on the previous manager, and on the very 'disturbed and disturbing' teenagers Homes were now having to cope with. In not going to see him and making sure that he knew all about the weekend's events, the staff on duty, without being fully aware they were doing it, were hoping to land him in the soup.

Soon after 9.30 a.m. one of them went to the general office to phone the two boys' social workers. Fairly detailed reports from the weekend out-of-hours social workers would already be awaiting the social workers when they came in – not usually before 9.30 a.m. on a Monday – but they would not have details of the boys' appalling behaviour when they got back from the police station. In telling the social workers, the residential care worker made sure that they understood that actually they couldn't cope with the boys in the Home. She implied that there would very soon be a formal request to remove them. A series of phone calls from the field work team, to the 'placements officer', to the service manager (Bob's manager) and to the assistant director for children and families, led to poor Bob receiving an irate phone call an hour later (just before he went into the kitchen to get his coffee) from the assistant director. He told Bob that he had no authority to request the removal of the two boys and that once young people had been placed at The Drive, then it was up to him and the staff to work with them. There was, he said, little point in having Homes if staff and managers were unwilling or unable to cope with children and young people for whom the department had to find accommodation. The assistant director had just started work on the following year's budget; he was being asked to make cuts of more than £1 million. Closing one of the three remaining children's Homes was one of his most favoured and straightforward contributions to this saving.

Bob was furious that someone had gone behind his back and asked for residents to be removed (which they hadn't), and he was also angry that he had been caught out so badly by knowing nothing of what had been going on at the weekend. He felt very foolish and recognised the barely disguised threat of closure in the assistant director's remarks.

However, before he had even left his office on the way to find the staff and sort out this problem, he was thinking to himself that closure might be the very best result from his point of view. The main thing would be to manage it well and come out of it with an excellent redundancy package; or to be moved, with his salary protected, into a job which suited him better.

Chapter 3

Noreen

Reg and Noreen are the owners and proprietors of a Home for adults with learning disabilities. It is called The Limes. They have built the Home up over many years. From very modest beginnings and with little experience of the work when they started in 1982, they have extended the building and the Home now has places for 18 residents, some of whom also have quite serious physical disabilities.

Reg is a builder. He is a director of the small building company which he founded and which is now run by his son. Noreen was a nurse and had worked with mentally handicapped people (as they were then described) in the local hospital before starting the Home. For many years, Noreen was also the 'matron' of the Home; later she called herself the manager. Last year, when she was 62, she decided to retire but she remains the joint proprietor with her husband and is still very fully involved in the Home. She and Reg appointed a 'care manager' who, after some problems, was 'registered' by the local authority inspection unit.

Today is the day of the first announced inspection since the care manager was appointed. Since 1992, when the Home had its first full inspection, Noreen has had her ups and downs with the inspection unit. Three different inspectors have visited and Noreen feels that they keep 'moving the goal posts'. She doesn't like inspections. To her, the system represents all the red tape and unnecessary interference so typical of the local authority, and the kind of rules-and-regulations mentality which she was so pleased to get away from when she left the hospital. She knew, at first hand, how abusive the hospital organisation often was to both patients and staff, and that each new crop of 'safeguards' was impossible to follow to the letter, and was there only to protect the management when something went wrong, as it inevitably did. In the early days of The Limes, when initially she had only eight residents and she worked all hours, helped by a couple of really excellent staff, the Home was truly a home. It was like 'one big family'. Two of the residents who came from the hospital in those early days of 'community care' (closing expensive hospitals) still live at the Home. They are now in their mid-seventies and The Limes is their true home. Three years ago, one of the inspectors realised that the Home was not registered for 'elderly people' but for 'adults' and required either that the older residents should now be moved to a suitable Home, or that The Limes had to apply for a different category of registration. It was not until Noreen had protested in the strongest possible terms and was preparing to lock the doors to any council official or social worker who dared to threaten the security of her older residents by, as she imagined, physically removing them from The Limes, that the chief inspector managed to make contact with her to tell her that including 'elderly people' in her registration was a very simple matter, and that it could be done with no disturbance, threat or disruption to the residents' lives. This was one issue on which there really was no need to consult them or in which they had to be involved in any way. It was essential to make the change to comply with the 1984 *Registered Homes Act*, which was there to protect residents from unscrupulous Home owners.

Noreen has never forgotten that crisis. She is still convinced that 'social services' could come into her Home and take residents away, and that it is only because she made such a fuss that they climbed down and the residents are still with her. She doesn't trust inspectors. They are 'inhuman, pen-pushing, little Hitlers'. She knows that there are some very poor Homes, and she is under no illusions about the motives of some of the other Home owners she meets at the local branch of their trade association; but the difference between them and her is so obvious that she is outraged by the apparent lack of perception on the part of inspectors, who should get on to those rotten Homes, where she knows there are all kinds of abuse going on. They should force them to improve or close them down and leave the good Homes, like The Limes, alone. That's what she would do.

A new inspector is doing this inspection and she's accompanied by a 'lay assessor', also new. There's been one of these lay assessors at each of the last two inspections, but they don't seem to do much, and they don't seem to know much about the residents or the work (rather like the inspectors themselves, in Noreen's opinion). Even though the new care manager, Thomas, is now well established and seems to be managing the Home very well, Noreen is determined to attend the inspection from start to finish. She is not going to let them get away with any nonsense and she doesn't want them upsetting Thomas, any of the staff or the residents. She's going to take notes, just as they do, so that she's got some evidence in case there's trouble afterwards.

Reg doesn't come to the Home every day but is very pleased with the success that Noreen has made of it. During the building slump, the Home has been a far more profitable business than the building firm, and has provided some useful work in building the large extension, in the steady addition of en-suite bathrooms to most of the bedrooms, in adapting the building for wheelchair access, and in regular maintenance. The Home is always well maintained and all the rooms are very regularly decorated to a high standard. Reg and his two employees are frequently in the Home, are known to all the residents, and are seen as very much part of the 'family'.

Noreen has found giving up the day-to-day management of the Home very difficult. Through hard work, instinctive and mostly excellent management, and through her firm grasp of practical principles, the Home has become a happy, thriving community where residents and staff enjoy life and work. Noreen has not been good at setting up all those systems which would prove to most inspectors that the Home does indeed work well. Many written procedures are still missing and those which have been provided have all been very grudgingly produced, and in Noreen's view are not worth the paper they are written on. It seems quite nonsensical to her that she has to spend valuable time producing policies and procedures whose only use is to be shown to inspectors. It reminds her of what her daughter, a teacher, says about school inspections. For this inspection she has actually put all these sheets of paper in frames and put them up in the dining room. That should shut the inspector up. She will take them down straight after the inspection because they spoil the look and atmosphere of the room.

Nearly all the staff share Noreen's common-sense distrust of and distaste for anything which professionalises and intellectualises giving good care. They follow the popular disdain for 'political correctness', and yet, for the most part, their approach to rights, dignity and self-determination – for residents and staff – is wholehearted and sincere. They just don't call it 'anti-oppressive' or 'anti-discriminatory practice'! Noreen's even heard it called 'ADP', which she thought was about as discriminatory as you could get and must have been invented by some college lecturer: another way to make sensible people feel excluded and foolish.

Noreen pays good wages and there are many other benefits attached to working at The Limes. Staff tend to stay a long time and are nearly always local. The Home is in a very mixed area – racially, culturally and economically – and the staff group reflect that mix; so do the residents. Noreen has never consciously tried to recruit a multiracial staff group; as she says, she just appoints the best people who apply. Initially she employed friends. In 1982, one of the two first care workers was a Jamaican friend from Noreen's Catholic church who had been working at another local care Home, and the other was a Sri Lankan colleague from the hospital. Both were about the same age as Noreen. The three of them had done everything in the Home at first; but gradually and without any formal structure being established, they became the *de facto* management team. Of course, Noreen was the registered manager and, as joint owner, she was taking some of the profits of the business, but the other two felt they had a considerable stake and were neither surprised nor particularly grateful when they were able to take substantial bonuses because annual profits were good.

As the Home expanded and the administrative burden became greater, as the complexities of organisation grew and the requirements from the inspection unit bore down on Noreen and her colleagues, the more they felt that 'the job isn't what it was'. When Noreen decided to retire from being the registered care manager, her two friends also retired, although they both remained very much involved as volunteers – visiting, arranging social events, and occasionally filling in for staff if for any reason there was a shortage.

Noreen and her friends think that the multiracial staff team which has been built up over the years is no more than a happy chance. They haven't made a conscious connection between the example set by the three of them and the way they work together and relate to each other. They would all say that a person's colour or culture – or age, religion or sexuality, for that matter – had nothing to do with their suitability for the job: they were selected simply on who was best. So having an equal opportunities policy, as required by the inspection unit and by the local authority when placing residents, seemed irrelevant to them. So often, they were far ahead of the cumbersome language of progressive policies and their earnest advocates who annoyed them so much; but in the face of this officious righteousness, they refused to analyse and understand how it was that they had achieved what the local authority itself and countless other employers were still striving, but failing, to achieve. Noreen felt demeaned by the clumsy questions and cold criticisms; in refusing to speak of her deep feelings and principles, she overreacted and portrayed herself as ignorant and incapable of thought.

There was much heart-searching and hard work in preparing to recruit to the new care manager's job. Noreen and Reg sought the help of the chief inspector, who, in spite of his position and supposed allegiances, they found to be a helpful and sympathetic person. He had gone out of his way to prevent the silly row about the registration categories from developing into a disaster. He showed his respect for the Home and the high quality of care provided, and although he supported the inspectors in all the requirements they made (indeed, as he pointed out, he read all reports and approved them before they went out), he freely admitted that he and his unit made mistakes sometimes, and, in retrospect he feels they could have handled that situation better. He was happy to help Noreen to think about how she should go about recruiting a care manager. He was clear about his duties and priorities; above all he wanted Homes of all kinds to give the best possible service. It was not only his job to monitor the quality of service, but also, whenever he could, to foster and promote it.

They advertised in *Community Care* and the *Guardian* as well as the local press. It cost them a fortune and Noreen couldn't believe that it would be worth it. The advertisement was unusual and honest. It said what the Home was like and it was clear about the person they wanted to fill the post: 'someone who can manage this Home through its next important, and difficult stage of development, and yet retain all the homeliness, informality, character and ideals of the Home as it is now'. Noreen was surprised by the result.

Fortunately the chief inspector had warned her that she might get a large number of replies, and that she might need to get some temporary help to send out application packs and then to process them when forms were returned. He also advised her to hire someone who was knowledgeable and skilled in the recruitment and selection of staff, to help with the person specification, the shortlisting and interviewing. The whole process cost Reg and Noreen thousands of pounds.

Thomas, an African man in his early forties, was the person selected by this time-consuming and expensive process in which residents and staff were included. He was a trained nurse, who, after working in several nursing and care Homes, had gained a Certificate in Social Service (CSS) – a two-year, generic qualification for social care. He had been officer in charge of a local authority Home for people with learning disabilities, and at the same time he had gained a Certificate in Management Studies (CMS).

The new care manager brought to The Limes professional knowledge and organised management skills, the lack of which were increasingly apparent as the Home grew larger and as Noreen and her colleagues became ever more exasperated with officialdom. But he was also very taken with the atmosphere of the Home as it was, and to him the challenge of this job was exactly as it had been stated in the advertisement. He was disillusioned with the local authority he had worked for because he put his principles above their short-term expediency. For example, he had refused to accept a client who was unsuitable for the Home and its group of residents. This was a man whose major problems were his mental illness and violent and threatening behaviour, who had been moved from the mental health hostel. Thomas also refused to accept staff who had been moved from other highly institutionalised settings when they were closed; and he refused to comply with instructions from the director of social services when he was ordered to do these things for he knew they would be detrimental to the well-being of residents and the long-term future of the Home. He was disciplined and he realised that the same situation would arise again sooner or later, and that next time he would be dismissed and, in all probability, the Home would be closed. He had lost all confidence in the management of the department; those whom he thought would support him vacillated and compromised, and Thomas began to look for another job. After careful discussion with him to understand his side of the story, his mixed, but in places damning, reference from his previous employers served only to recommend Thomas to his new employers at The Limes, though it caused the inspection unit to delay his registration as care manager.

Thomas has been at The Limes for about six months by the day of the inspection. Of course, he is well aware of the sixteen requirements and sixty-seven recommendations made in the last report. Knowing that the Home could not comply with all the requirements and follow all the recommendations – some of which were not sensible – he began to renegotiate them with the inspector. After the last inspection Noreen had got to the stage of deliberately ignoring the inspection unit – or, rather, this particular inspector; and the inspector had responded to Noreen in an equally pig-headed fashion. It took a visit from Thomas to the inspector, and some behind-the-scenes intervention on the part of the chief inspector (who felt that he should have identified and challenged the impasse which was developing) to begin turning around the very negative relationship which was becoming so dangerously entrenched. In a new job, with new-found authority and confidence, and away from his own sad experience of confrontation with a domineering organisation, Thomas felt his considerable skills of negotiation were suddenly available. He found it delightfully easy to get on very positive terms with the inspectors and to agree a realistic programme of development based on the needs of residents, rather than on the antagonisms and authoritarianism which had been inherent in the relationship before.

Thomas has been looking forward to the inspection. He has done a lot of work with Noreen and the staff to help them to be more open, and to assure them that the really important things at The Limes are done well. 'It is a very good place. Inspections can be helpful: they can highlight the positives (of which there are many), and, by being knowledgeable outsiders, they can identify things which need improvement; they can ask the questions which insiders don't ask. They have also got an important, legitimate job to do, and it's in all our and residents' interests that they do it well.'

Thomas has got a long way with the staff but Noreen is more difficult to convince. She still comes in on the day of the inspection, ready to do battle and defend the Home against attack.

The inspection goes very well. Thomas manages it with delicacy and humour. The inspector relaxes; the lay assessor is fascinated to hear Thomas talking about the work; even Noreen finds herself agreeing with the inspector on occasions. Instead of defending the indefensible with increasingly ridiculous arguments and accusing the inspector of ignorance and inexperience, she is discussing issues and differences of perception. The inspector never gets into an inquisitorial mode of operation nor does she threaten. When she's making notes, it's quite clear what she's making notes about. Noreen soon forgets her resolution to note everything herself in preparation for the battles to come.

At the end of the inspection, they all meet together. The inspector is highly complimentary and encouraging about the Home. She tells them clearly and simply what requirements and recommendations she is likely to make, and these come as no surprise because they have all been discussed during the inspection.

Noreen can't believe that the experience could be so different. She is delighted but remains a little suspicious. She rings Reg after the inspectors have gone: 'Perhaps the report will be like all the others and this was just a different presentation on the part of the inspectors? But one thing's for sure, Thomas knows what he's doing. He handled them like a dream. For the first time, I know I've done the right thing to retire. We needed a pro in this job, and we've found one.'

Thomas writes a few quick notes. He goes round to see staff and residents to tell them how it went, and by 7 p.m. he's on his way home. A good day's work, but hard. And the hardest work of all was Noreen!

Chapter 4

Lok

Lok is the manager of the local authority's residential and day care services for older people. He is known as the 'service manager'. The authority used to have twelve Homes and five day centres, but in the last few years since *Community Care* (the Act) and the pressure to cut the department's budget these have dwindled down to five Homes and two day centres. The residential Homes were always the most expensive service, and the councillors were prepared to face the temporary protests provoked by their closure in order to achieve such large chunks of saving at one go. Neighbouring local authorities had gone even further and one was left with no Homes of its own at all.

Of the Homes previously run by the local authority, one is now managed by a private company; three are run by a housing association; and three have been shut altogether. One of the day centres which was closed by the council was then reopened by a local voluntary organisation to care for people with dementia. It has now closed again because referrals have dried up and the local authority will not agree a sufficiently long-term contract to enable improvements to be made or for adequate levels of staff to be employed. Everyone agrees that more day care provision for older people with dementia is essential but there isn't the money to pay for it.

Lok is managing a service under siege. As Homes and day centres have been closed, most staff in them have been given the option of jobs in the remaining establishments, the managers of which have had no choice but to accept them. If there's a vacancy, it is filled by a worker from a closed establishment. As the service shrinks, the staff withdraw behind the inner walls. It is like the siege of a medieval castle. Supplies are running out and everything within the castle becomes hugely expensive. The population and the army know they are doomed; they fight amongst themselves and their spirits are as low as they could be. They see the enemy outside looking happy, well-fed and free. There are constant defections. Those in command are hated. All anyone has to look forward to is the end of the siege.

Lok has the misfortune to be in command of this particular castle – the service. Every year new cuts are proposed and parts of the service are chopped. The 'papers' which Lok and his manager (the assistant director) present to councillors describe these cuts as 'restructuring'; the popular business phrase 're-engineering' is also creeping into the council's management vocabulary. The proposals are always couched in the most optimistic terms and look forward to 'productive partnerships' with the 'independent sector'. (In this context, 'independent' means any organisation which is not directly controlled by the council.) However, the local voluntary organisation which had to give up running the day centre was anything but independent; it was in fact totally dependent on the council. The small, privately run Homes are dependent on the fees paid and, in effect, set by the council: fees which are far below the costs of places in the local authority Homes. As the council virtually dictates the fees it pays, Home owners pare down their costs – most frequently by reducing staffing levels and wages. The inspectors then require them to restore adequate staffing levels, and some of them end up trying to steer a very narrow course between financial ruin on one side because the council will not pay adequate fees, and, on the other side, having their registration cancelled because they cannot meet required standards. The council forces the 'independent sector' to make the savings and to pay wages which it cannot get away with itself. The council would argue, with justification, that the government has done the same to them, forcing local authorities to administer an underfunded service.

Nevertheless Lok would like a job with one of the larger independent-sector organisations. He doesn't much mind if it is a private or voluntary organisation, just so long as it isn't directly controlled by the local authority. He is trying to establish good contacts with all the organisations the council works with. He has been with this department for five years, coming as one of two managers in the days just before the big cuts began. He had been a middle-ranking administrator in social services in a neighbouring authority, had been seconded to a Certificate of Qualification in Social Work (CQSW) course and from there had become an 'adult Homes manager' for the same department. For all of the twenty-five years he had worked in Britain, he had been known to colleagues as 'Luke' because people had found it difficult to use his Vietnamese name. (It was not as if it was difficult to say; it was more because it just wouldn't 'do' as a name.) Everyone, from director to care assistant, knew him as Luke. His surname was never used. He felt it was far too late and too difficult to change this now. It was, he considered, the least of his problems – if it was a problem at all.

Lok's current most pressing problem is with the manager, staff and even the residents of one of the Homes. They appear to be in revolt.

Four years earlier, as part of the 'new deal' involving a first wave of major cuts and closures, this Home – Norwood House – was converted, at great expense, into a 'resource centre'. This meant that it would have four 'group living units' (one specialising in caring for people with dementia), a respite care unit, a day centre and a luncheon club. In addition there would be all sorts of social, recreational, cultural, health, education and entertainment facilities, and events for both resident and non-resident pensioners. Norwood House was reopened with a flourish after nearly two years of conversion work. The residential units (including the respite care unit) still provided places for up to seventy-five residents, at a cost of something over £350 per week for each residential place. The overall annual cost, before any income was taken into account, was approximately £1.5 million – of which day care accounted for less than 10 per cent.

Initially Norwood House was a great success. With a new manager and an injection of fresh and enthusiastic staff making up independent but closely coordinated teams for each residential unit and each of the other services, there was a liveliness and vigour which, for once, meant that the place genuinely did what the hype had said that it would do.

The Home served its locality (which is what the council had said it was going to do). It was a good place to visit, to live in and to work in. For local people it was a focus, and was excellent for the council's public relations: here at last was something which the council was doing well.

It seemed odd, however, that it was not universally popular within the social services department and the council as a whole. People working in the other Homes found the attention which Norwood House attracted, and the additional resources which they assumed it was given, particularly irksome, when they were struggling to do the same job with so much less recognition and support. This did not spur them on to emulate Norwood House, but to wish to undermine and destroy it. In fact the weekly 'unit cost' (how much each place cost per week) was much higher in most of the other Homes. This was partly because they were smaller but mostly because of unnecessarily high staffing costs (with a lot of overtime and agency fees caused by understaffing, absenteeism and sickness) and relatively low occupancy (they were not attractive Homes to live in, and there were better options, including Norwood House).

The manager of Norwood House had taken her brief very seriously and was determined to make a success of the new venture. At the time of her appointment one of the 'management development initiatives' in the department had been to flatten the hierarchy, to establish 'cost centres' and devolve budgets and decision-making. There were also attempts to divide the department into 'purchasing' and 'providing' sections. As the department 'downsized' it became obvious that the administrative and managerial staff at headquarters needed reducing even more than those staff who either assessed 'customers' and 'purchased' a service on their behalf, or those who 'provided' a service, like the residential Homes. So the section in which Lok worked was halved, leaving him as the sole service manager.

While Rachel, the manager of Norwood House, tried to use these developments to improve the service and increase both choice and control for residents and other users of the resource centre, nearly every-one else in the department – especially those who had been working there for some time – saw the changes only as attacks on their jobs. They had seen changes like this before, and each time they had fought them, gained a few temporary concessions, and lost. The council would be more honest if it simply called all this preposterous window dressing 'cuts . . . and more cuts'. They felt that Rachel was either naive or a management tool.

Some of the things which had been going on at Norwood House provoked union displeasure. Some staff were happily taking on respon-sibilities which were not in their job descriptions. The demarcation between jobs, often a barrier to good care in other Homes, was almost disappearing at Norwood House. Staff didn't take regular and set breaks. They made arrangements between themselves about who would do which jobs, and when they would have their lunch or coffee breaks. If there wasn't time, they just didn't take the break. (In fact it was just the same in some of the other Homes – the better ones – but they kept it quiet, and when under pressure – from the management or their unions – they reverted to the rules.) Staff acting as key workers did the job as if they were the equal of care managers (on the 'purchasing side'); they would even take the lead in making decisions about admissions. They refused to have any agency staff in the Home. Everyone had induction and regular supervision. It was no longer possible to talk solely with the manager about an admission; she would refer applicants to the team leaders of the units which had vacancies. All staff and some residents and neighbourhood users of the centre attended a big meeting every fortnight. This meeting was treated as the most important decision-making forum, and acted as if it could question or even overturn decisions made by the social services management and the union. People working at Norwood House behaved as if they were a law unto themselves. Their stance questioned the authority and power of the old bosses: unions and management.

Of course, Rachel maintained that they were putting the 'management development initiative' into practice, and Lok was caught in the middle of an increasingly tense situation. While he agreed with what was happening at Norwood House and knew that their widely recognised success (mostly outside the department) reflected well on him too, he was seen by his managers as being insufficiently in control. The senior managers regarded Rachel and her colleagues as headstrong and requiring firm management. Some of her principles were impractical, and even if they did appear in her own job description and in the proclaimed plans for the new resource centre, every hard-headed manager has to compromise given the harsh realities of rapidly changing circumstances. In the opinion of the director and assistant director (Lok's manager), not to compromise was to betray an underlying unsuitability for the job.

When Lok first came to work for the department – on his very first day – he had unwittingly crossed a picket line. He was very worried that if he didn't comply with his first day's instructions, he might get off to a very bad start with his managers. When he reached the main door of the building, there was a line of about ten people, holding banners, who handed him leaflets and chanted something about ambulance drivers. With his mind set on the tricky business of starting work for a new employer, and not for a moment thinking that he was doing anything of great importance or lasting significance, he politely took the leaflets and walked past the demonstrators into the building. Lok found it almost deserted. Very few people had crossed the picket line. It was only later that, sitting in the empty personnel section, unable to comply with his first day's instructions for starting work, he looked at the leaflets. Lok discovered that it was a day's strike called on behalf of the social services transport section whose work was about to be put out to tender. This innocent misdemeanour was never forgotten.

Although he joined the union, he rarely found himself in sympathy with its local leaders. Yet he knew that his manager got on very well with them, and it seemed to him that, in the case of Norwood House, they were at one in their attempts to bring it into line. It felt as if every-one was playing a game. They were fierce enemies, in opposing teams, while the game was on, but they drank together and slapped each other on the back in the bar after the game. Give them a common enemy and they would joyously combine to 'kick his head in'. If you didn't or couldn't join in this (mostly male) camaraderie, you were thought to be a bit odd, and were in danger of being picked on at some point. It astounded Lok that half these people were trained social workers, and had spent considerable time learning about social psychology and organisational and group behaviour.

In his five years in this local authority, Lok had never really felt accepted. He was 'in' with neither the management nor the union. He was not a part of the various social groupings and 'sets' within his workplace. Although he was proud of and at ease with his ethnicity within himself, he felt excluded by the White racism which, despite all protestations to the contrary, was woven into the fabric of this organisation; yet he also felt unwelcome in the Black workers' and managers' groups in which people had successfully joined together both to support each other and to bring about change in the organisation. There were women's groups and lesbian and gay groups, formal and informal, which were also active and supportive, but even if Lok had been eligible for membership by sex or sexuality, he would not have joined. He was not a 'joiner'; nor was he a loner – he just did not feel the need to define himself and be in a 'club'. In some ways, he reflected, this organisation was a collection of separate, exclusive, competing, groups and factions. The potential of all these different people joining together in a common endeavour (social service) was enormous – but frightening. He watched his colleagues duck away from the responsibility of their real task and it appeared as if for much of the time they had forgotten their common purpose; they were intent only on their survival and supremacy in an untrusting and threatening world. Their world, in the headquarters of the social services department, was a comparatively well paid, even a comparatively secure, physically comfortable environment. Though privileged, however, it was a spiritually impoverished position. How could such an organisation provide reliable services to people who were economically and physically weak and vulnerable?

Lok knew that something was happening at Norwood House which modelled and embodied the purposefulness, the cohesiveness, the direct provision of real practical help, the inclusion and celebration of differences amongst people, which the organisation proclaimed it stood for – but of which it was most fearful. Lok was on his own both in his perception and through his exclusion. Had he joined any group, he would have to pay the price – his membership fee – of subscribing to the 'group view', of seeing things from one particular angle.

He was now worried that, even though it was embodying high professional and ethical values, Norwood House itself had no alternative in this organisation other than to become another faction, fighting for survival and supremacy.

Today Lok is going to meet with Rachel. He takes with him this clear organisational view, his commitment to Norwood House and high professional values, his awareness of the pressures all around (the siege mentality), his hopes of finding a job elsewhere, his strong sense of justice combined with a measure of fatalism – and he takes with him his orders from his boss: 'Sort them out, Luke. Get control. Or they're next for the chop.' (In Lok's mind, he distinctly heard this overbearing and insensitive man, the assistant director, add 'Chop chop, old chap.' But his boss had learned not to say such things – only to think them and laugh to himself. He was too stupidly arrogant to sense that Lok might hear his thoughts without his speaking them.)

Chapter 5

Janet and Jeeva

Janet is the director of care services for a large housing association. She has been in the job for three years. After graduating from university, doing Voluntary Service Overseas, and working for two years with a charity helping people living on the streets, Janet became a housing officer for a housing association. She then worked as a local authority housing officer before returning to a housing association as a 'supported housing manager'. In that capacity she managed the teams supporting tenants in their own flats and two registered care Homes for more dependent people who had previously lived in long-term wards in psychiatric hospitals.

When Janet arrived at the Hetherington Housing Trust, the organisation was already widely involved in residential care, although in most schemes it did not directly manage the provision of care.

Housing associations have unique access to capital and revenue from the Housing Corporation, and many of them have eagerly filled the gaps caused by closures of the long-stay hospitals and by the local authorities' rush to get out of residential care. In some ways they are suitable organisations to have done so, but in others they are not. There are two principal underlying problems. First, that this development has been partly driven by the ambitions of senior staff to expand their organisation and thereby expand their own jobs and status (and salaries!). Second, that they know very little about residential care and its management. (Of course, in neither problem are they alone; the ambition of so many senior managers in social care organisations, and their appetite for power and influence, combined with their ignorance, have always been the curse of residential work.)

The results of this eager move into a new area of work, which is not primarily a housing task, are very mixed. Most of the contracts are far from straightforward. The funding is complex, and it is common for managers and staff in residential and nursing Homes) not to know which organisation is truly responsible for them. All the management and funding arrangements have been negotiated and agreed with little or no reference to them, and neither they nor the residents were consulted while the wheeling and dealing was going on. The process bears an unpleasant resemblance to the operations in which large private companies buy and sell small firms and works, incorporating them, disposing of them and swapping them around, often for tactical and short-term financial gain. The arrangements of housing associations and their 'business' partners are so complicated that even those who are making the deals are frequently unsure of exactly what new agreements they are signing up to. Residents and staff are left powerless and confused – and often angry. The promise of a reliable, concerned, accessible, responsive managing organisation – the sort of organisational context required for high-quality care – is too frequently broken. Managers negotiating deals between the housing associations, local authorities, health authorities and health service trusts forget that the spoiled broth which they cook up between them is what staff and residents in Homes have to consume. (Too often, that image of providing food can be taken literally. Some housing associations have 'contracted out' catering in Homes to catering companies, or to the catering services of local authorities or health service trusts. By thus detaching from 'home life' one of its most central and significant aspects they rip the heart out of a Home.)

Even with her limited experience of residential care, Janet knew that standards in most of the twenty-four registered care Homes and four nursing Homes which came within her 'care services' division were barely adequate. A small number of the Homes were outstandingly good. There were about six different management contracts and arrangements, and most of them were unclear, even to Janet.

Janet wanted to know what it was that made the few Homes work well. On the face of it, it wasn't the management contract because only two of the Homes which worked well were managed by the same arrangements. However, the Homes which worked well did all come under the same care services manager (the post between Janet and the head of Home or care manager) and comprised nearly half the Homes he managed.

So one ingredient in the success of these Homes could be his way of managing. Jeeva, the service manager, was the only person in her division with real experience of residential care, both as a care worker and as a manager. He was also an enthusiast who believed that living in a Home could be a very positive choice for people, and that the work itself was intellectually and emotionally demanding, and, when done well, was a very satisfying job. Although he was well organised and highly competent, Jeeva never allowed the financial and administrative management of his group of Homes to dominate his work. He always seemed to have time to talk with people and was totally reliable in his visits to the Homes, his supervision with managers, and holding regular meetings. And he obviously enjoyed his work.

At the same time Jeeva was an outspoken critic of the various management arrangements. Although in some ways he was proving the contrary, he maintained that it was impossible to provide good care when there were so many, mostly very inefficient, organisations involved. He complained that he (as named 'person in control' representing the housing association) had no real power to carry out his responsibilities. In one Home where an inspection report had insisted that the kitchen floor must be replaced, he had to inform the health service trust (contracted to run the Home) who, only when they had budgeted for the cost of the work, told the local authority works department (with which they had a maintenance and building contract for the building), who, in turn, and after surveying and costing the work itself, gave the work to a private building firm with whom they had a contract for minor building and maintenance work. (This was a firm which, ironically, the housing association itself also used.) The replacement of the kitchen floor took two years, and Jeeva reckoned that the real costs of administrative and management time far exceeded the cost of the work. But, as he pointed out, the cost was not the biggest problem. The inspectors had, rightly, said the floor was dangerous. Residents and staff were at risk throughout the two-year period, and Jeeva felt foolish and impotent, as did the Home's care manager.

In another Home the care manager had pointed out to Jeeva that it was seriously understaffed. He agreed but told the care manager that she should take up the issue with her employers, the health service trust, who were contracted with the housing association to provide 'adequate staffing'. She had already done so. In the employer's view the Home was 'adequately staffed'; it had always been staffed at that level before the housing association took over responsibility for running the Home. In any case the health service trust said they could not afford to staff it more fully. Yet an inspection report to the 'person in control' (Jeeva) required that the staffing ratios should be increased.

After eighteen months of negotiations, the local health authority and social services (who jointly funded residents at the Home) agreed to pay the health services trust a higher fee, in order that the health services trust could pay the housing association a higher management charge, in order that they in turn could pay the trust the higher staffing costs involved. The arrangement was unbelievably cumbersome, wasteful and stupid (it had also been suggested that it was illegal), and yet it had been negotiated and signed up to by the three senior managers involved, including Janet's predecessor. Of course, such arrangements (which are still common throughout the service) meant that it was very difficult to establish whose responsibility anything at all was. In the event of a catastrophe, it was far more likely that Jeeva or the care manager would be forced to take responsibility – after all, they were the registered names – than would any of the senior managers who were so indifferent to the results of their grand but foolish arrangements. Janet was determined to change this.

The contracts for care were drawn up with many different organisations, but they all had their near-incomprehensibility in common. They were appallingly written, abounding in phrases such as 'to provide a responsive environment', 'the frail elderly', 'care facilities ensuring opportunities to socialise and access to appropriate therapeutic activities'. Not only was the language inaccessible and nonsensical, but the content displayed a deep ignorance of the principles and practice of residential care and its management. For instance, in many contracts there appeared the sentence: 'Where rooms are shared, the residents will be able to choose their own companions.' Janet knew that this was simply not the case. The 'voluntary' sharing of rooms between people who were not partners or had not initially asked to share a room with a particular friend or family member (for whatever reason didn't matter) was a sham. None of the people writing or signing up to this policy had imagined *themselves* in this situation, and this thoroughly dishonest statement exposed their disconnectedness from the realities of living in a residential Home. The whole tone of these documents was obscure and élitist, and yet Janet reflected that she had somehow got caught up in this way of thinking and behaving.

When she sometimes found herself thinking about how she started working in social care (doing voluntary service and working with homeless people who were living on the streets) and about her ideals at the time, Janet regretted how far she had got away from all that. Now she was a 'senior manager'; she earned a very good salary; she had a car and a house and, although she worked hard, she lived a life which had little connection with the lives of the association's 'service users' (another 'contract language' phrase to distance and sanitise real people) and with the staff who worked directly with them – and earned a quarter of what she was paid. Of course, she gave generously to people begging on the street, and would argue their case strongly to friends she was with, who might ask her why she gave so freely. As she would say, 'I once worked with those people; I know what their lives are like.' Of course, she bought the *Big Issue* regularly, but she was beginning to question herself more about what she really was doing in this job. She felt she was now caught up in a culture which, earlier in her life, she had despised and had thought she was fighting to change.

Janet had arranged to get some independent supervision in the last six months. Although she received (and insisted on receiving) supervision from the chief executive of the association every month, it tended to be very 'business' orientated, leaving little time for thinking and reflection. Her job was like that: rushing from one meeting to another, arriving at work early and staying late, preparing committee reports and making complicated bids to other organisations.

The work grew and grew, yet Janet felt that what she did was having less and less effect on what her part of the organisation was there to do – to look after people, to support them, to give care, or, as the annual report would say, to 'deliver services'.

Janet met regularly with Jeeva and the other two service managers. They had a meeting together fortnightly and she also held individual supervision sessions with them every two weeks. In the two years that he had been working with her, Jeeva had never missed a meeting or supervision. He was always enthusiastic about both. With Jeeva's lively and sometimes controversial contributions at the meetings, and his insistence on using his supervision sessions as times to work at knotty issues of professional development as well as reporting on work in progress, Janet often felt challenged and yet satisfied by their contact. When she was in Jeeva's company she knew that the job could be worth doing. He had the knack of never making her feel either superior to him or undermined by him. His prime interest was absolutely clear – giving the very best service to residents – and his open enthusiasm and energy were infectious.

Janet had learned a lot about Jeeva's successful style of management, and about the principles and attitudes which underpinned the style. The people he worked with trusted him. He could always be relied on to say what he thought and believed. Jeeva didn't indulge in moaning and whining about his criticisms of the organisation; he just voiced them and he was open about wishing to make improvements. Once Janet had got used to this, she found it stimulating, but her colleagues, the other directors and members of the management committee and subcommittees, viewed Jeeva as arrogant. They dismissed him as a know-all and, without finding out that the staff in the Homes had a good opinion of him, assumed that his management style was high-handed, interfering and too 'hands on' – the very opposite of the reality experienced by those with whom he worked so well. Janet also suspected (and Jeeva knew) that part of their antipathy to him was that he was gay. They had been so pleased to appoint a Mauritian as a middle manager – his photo looked good in the annual report – but when Jeeva did nothing to conceal his sexuality, they felt somehow cheated. Provoked by his professional and personal candour, their instincts were to attempt to 'rein him in' and to bring him in line with the other managers at his level. Janet's instincts told her differently. Knowing the real value of Jeeva's work and observing the consistently high standards and the new developments in the Homes which he managed, Janet began to think that Jeeva would be the key to making the radical changes in management which she knew were needed.

On an official visit to one of the nursing Homes, Janet had been shocked by an incident she witnessed (pp. 186–95). When she raised her concerns with Jeeva, he had shown her how she had completely misread the situation, although, he reassured her, all outsiders would have seen it the way she had done unless they really understood how the minutiae of residential care fitted into a whole picture.

By agreement with Jeeva and the heads of some of the Homes in his group, Janet began spending time in the Homes. She felt she needed to understand what exactly it was that she was managing and for which she took overall responsibility. To begin with, when she visited at the weekends, or early in the morning or after work in the evenings, although staff and residents in these Homes were very welcoming, at heart they felt as if she was testing them out and 'inspecting' them. There were many things she didn't understand. With her experience of working with a wide variety of homeless people, she had thought that she would not find spending time in a Home too difficult, and she was surprised by just how challenging it was. Often she didn't know what to do – how to handle a situation – and yet a care assistant would come along and respond to the resident in question with such practised ease and sensitivity that Janet was left wondering whether, in her earlier direct work with clients, she herself had ever achieved such a level of skill.

She found it interesting and revealing that residents in the Homes she visited were not in the slightest bit impressed or overawed when she explained her position as director of care services. Most residents were not at all interested in the technicalities of the complex organisational relationships, negotiations and contracts which took up so much of Janet's time and energy. For them, the important and influential people in the organisation were 'their' staff and the manager of the Home (whose official title was nursing team leader). In these Homes, they did not imagine that there was anyone who really told the head of Home what to do – apart from them. They knew Jeeva and liked him a lot, but they did not see him as 'the boss' or the man from 'head office'; he was just a frequent visitor who had regular meetings with the care manager and some of the staff, and was always happy to stop and talk. He was useful in that when he attended residents' and relatives' meetings, he was sometimes able to find ways of providing extra resources, and he knew other Homes which were prepared to lend or share some of their resources. However, neither Jeeva's nor Janet's actual position was of any interest or consequence to most of the residents whom Janet got to know through her visits.

Having got to know more about the work in the Homes, and when she had begun to enjoy her visits more, Janet arranged a series of meetings with Jeeva to discuss the possibilities for radical change in the care services division.

Janet wanted to start planning straight away, partly because she was aware of the housing association committee 'cycle' which would determine how quickly any plans could be agreed and implemented. But she was also worried about the impending annual negotiations over the 'care contracts' under which the association bought the staffing for several Homes from two different community care health service trusts. The two nursing Homes which she had spent time in and which Jeeva managed for the housing association had a comprehensive contract for 'care and hotel services' (the latter involving cleaning, catering, laundry, etc.) with one of these trusts.

Jeeva managed four residential Homes which were staffed by another trust but where 'hotel services' were provided by yet another trust, which then subcontracted the maintenance to a local authority! Much as he disagreed with the complex mess of the management arrangements, Jeeva had found a way of working with all the staff teams which had improved the care immensely. He felt that both the nursing Homes were ready to move into a further stage of development which a clearer and more autonomous form of management could help to bring about. Already the real managers of the Homes (currently called the nursing team leaders) felt that Jeeva was there to help, support and give management supervision, not to direct. (This was in spite of the fact that the nursing team leaders' 'line' manager was a general manager in the health service trust.) They were now keen to take on more of the full management responsibilities of the Homes, and with Jeeva's encouragement they were doing so. As good managers often have to do, he was making a bad system work by involving people both in adaptations and in developing a real understanding of the system, which then helped them not to be totally constrained by it. Having spent some time in these two nursing Homes, and knowing Jeeva's views of the existing management arrangements, Janet was now very keen to make big changes. To Janet's surprise and annoyance, Jeeva was not so enthusiastic.

Although he knew that the staff in both Homes were ready to make changes (and were already making them), he was worried that neither of the managing organisations involved in this contract was ready to make the changes required. (Of the two, he was more concerned about the housing association than the health service trust, because it would be taking on additional commitments.) Jeeva felt that organisations which had got themselves entangled in such a silly contract in the first place, had continued to renew them year after year, and had been hostile to the adaptations which he, the nursing team leaders and the staff teams had made, had not yet done the preparatory work necessary to make such changes. Their first step towards getting themselves ready to change would be to become aware of how obstructive the contract was to giving a good service, and to acknowledge their own complicity and responsibility.

Jeeva admired the way that Janet had set about her own 'conversion' and underestimated neither its importance nor Janet's key role in developing the service along the lines which he would like to see. But her 'conversion' was fairly recent, and he knew that fundamental and sustainable change was rarely brought about by the immediate implementation of 'bright ideas', however strongly inspired. He and Janet were part of a large organisation, and while he had found ways of resisting, avoiding and even working with the organisational pressures and yet still managing changes in the service, he knew there was a lot of work yet to be done if one obstructive system of management was not going to be replaced by another which was equally flawed.

Janet had been incensed by seeing how badly the 'care contract' was working for residents. She saw how, in giving away its control of staffing, the housing association had no way of stopping the use of 'bank' and agency staff, or even the removal of key members of the teams to go and work elsewhere in the trust's other Homes or hospitals.

Janet knew that Jeeva had tried to stop this sort of practice, and that the team leader had also confronted her line manager in the trust about it, but it was still happening. But in spite of Janet's anger and determination that such things would not happen if the housing association were to manage staff directly, Jeeva knew that she did not yet fully understand the complexities and the organisational demands of staffing the Homes in the way she undoubtedly wished them to be staffed. The housing association would have to employ more staff and they would have to hand over full responsibility to the manager and the team. On neither count was Janet yet ready to accept the implications of change. But this was a hard message for Jeeva to convey, even though Janet had great trust in his experience and judgement and was, as he recognised, remarkably open and self-aware.

Part II

Thinking about residential care: its context, organisation and management

Chapter 6

The wider picture and the core task

What is management? – Managing to what end? – Getting away from the primary task – The design of a suitable organisation

Throughout the examples set out in Part I we have seen the contrast between two sorts of management. One is represented by Marcia, Thomas, Rachel and Jeeva – people who organise resources, who know what their jobs are, who have a constant awareness of the context in which they work, and who *get things done*. For them managing is an integral part of their work; they do not move from 'managing' to 'doing' and back again; they do not recognise a separation yet they are clear about their own boundaries of responsibility. The other sort of management is represented by Marcia's manager, by Bob and by the senior managers in most of the organisations portrayed in these examples. They are managers for whom management itself has become the objective rather than part of a process or a means to an end. The primary task is forgotten and the organisation flounders in the morass created by their struggles for self-preservation and aggrandisement. Lok is caught in the middle of the two types of management, and Janet, as a senior manager, is attempting to get back to doing what she originally came into this type of work to do.

In this chapter we consider why this subversion of the task occurs, and how organisations can be redesigned and managed to carry out the primary task of residential care.

WHAT IS MANAGEMENT?

As a process, management is the organisation required to get a job done. The structure of such management has the person doing the job at its centre, though it takes in the wider picture to include as part of management all those people and resources that surround, support, coordinate and monitor the work of that central figure.

But in the last thirty years, management, both as an activity and as a structure, has been embellished by pretentious and superior notions which have split managing from doing. Even twenty years ago, the word 'management' was not much used in social care organisations. Seniority, advanced training, expertise and good organisation were no less essential but were seen to be integral to accomplishing the task. Now the widely accepted view of management as a structure is of a whole organisation with the most senior manager, the director or chief executive, at the top. In this picture, the people who carry out the task – who do the job – and the customers or clients of the service are peripheral. They lose their significance. In discussion about the organisation, they will occupy a very small proportion of people's attention, even if they figure as comforting figures in the organisation's publicity.

Whose creation is such a view? It is certainly not the view seen by either the client or the person who does the job for the client. They are both likely to be ignorant of or confused by this fanciful construction which appears in the annual report or is depicted in the organisational chart. Such productions are grandiose fantasies bearing little resemblance to how the organisation actually works. And yet this picture – this conceptualisation – becomes the organisation and defines its management. Even though we know it is unreal, we accept it as the way things are – and always will be.

MANAGING TO WHAT END?

The effects of subverting the primary task

What clients want is a worker or a team of workers who can give them the care that they need (see Chapter 8). Providing that service – meeting that need – is the objective of a care organisation. The primary task – the *raison d'être* – should be self-evident in any contact at the point where the service is given. Clients have no reason to be interested in the grand, complicated construction which planners, managers, consultants, chief executives and committee members have dreamed up. Few clients and basic-grade staff know the difference between the immediate line manager of the part of the organisation with which they deal, and the chief executive; it doesn't matter to them. The absurd aggrandisement of the organisation will come to their notice and be of concern to them only if they become aware of the gulf between the service they receive and the service they are supposed to receive according to the organisation's public declaration of intent when promoting its image.

Examples abound of conflicting messages, clashing motives, unclear purposes and of the harm done by splitting managing from doing. They are part of our shared, contemporary British experience of organisations and their management, whether in welfare services or privatised utilities. When British Gas was proclaiming that the company was giving a vastly improved service, issuing all sorts of guarantees and promises, boasting of a 'charter mark' and publicly rewarding its most senior staff with vast salaries and bonuses, many individual customers became aware of, and increasingly angry about, the gap between the puff and the real performance. They could not help comparing the glossy advertising and self-congratulatory statistics with their real experience of shoddy service and inaccurate bills (Peter Lennon, 14 December 1996, *Guardian*). Similarly, Yorkshire Water became very unpopular when it failed to fulfil what customers had always assumed was its primary task – providing water. Unfortunately, some customers had missed the significant difference between the primary task of a publicly owned utility and that of a money-making business. The old primary task of providing water became merely the means by which the privatised company would achieve its new core objective – to make profits for its shareholders.

It may be assumed, and inferred from their performance, that the very highly paid managers of such companies also have an individual core objective which is to make large amounts of money for themselves. Under these sorts of pressures and the demands of very different primary tasks, care of the customer becomes merely a matter of commercial judgement. Such companies will now ask, 'Will this improvement in service and customer care increase profits?'

Social care organisations, and residential care in particular, whose primary task at first sight truly is care of the customer, are subject to the same pressures of greed and aggrandisement, of hunger for power, money and status as are those commercial companies which social care organisations increasingly try to imitate. It is interesting that among some of the better organisations providing social care are those which, as money-making businesses, do ask the question, 'Will this improvement in care increase profits?' For good commercial care companies the answer is usually 'yes'; other less successful, 'down-market' (and often smaller) private providers are forced to answer 'no' to the same question (see p. 28). Thus the gap grows between the more expensive care and accommodation provided to customers able to afford such Homes, and the barely or sometimes less than adequate Homes which are dependent on residents who are unable to pay for their own care.

Identifying and clarifying the primary task

Clarifying the primary task is the first act of management at every level. The manager must ask herself or himself, 'What is this organisation here to do, and what is my part in it?'. If the task is unclear, or if the task is found to be different at different levels or in different departments of the organisation, the service will deteriorate and the client will suffer. In a 'not for profit' organisation, the basic-grade worker or the domestic assistant must share the same overall primary task as the chief executive. The primary task will be communicated to clients by the service they receive from the basic-grade worker, and it is on the standard of that service that the chief executive should be judged.

The big care companies

In the commercial world of private care providers, the primary task will be to maximise profits for the shareholders and/or proprietors, but because care is the company business, the way in which it makes its profits, only those companies providing a high-quality service at a competitive price will attract customers. At least, that is the theory. However, in a genuinely competitive market, this entails the demise of some private providers and a fluidity in the whole range of private provision as some companies fail; or as they prosper and take over other ailing companies; and as new companies enter the market. As an employee in a private company, the only way in which a worker can share the same primary task as the owner or chief executive is by being given a financial stake in the company profits. Some companies have the foresight to do this.

Of course, very few care companies declare their true primary task to the customer or to their care-giving employees. They could argue that since making a profit has to be the aim of any private business, there is no need to 'declare' it in this way. They are more likely to say that their primary task is providing care rather than to acknowledge that this is the means by which they make a profit. But neither the customer nor the employee is likely to be fooled by this, any more than customers of

Sainsbury's or Tesco's believe that these companies' sole reason for existence is to provide as many people as possible with the best-quality food at the lowest price. If that was their primary objective, they would have no reason not to collaborate in achieving it rather than to undercut, outsell and beat the other into second place. Both companies exist to make profits; their means of achieving these profits may be, in part, by beating their competitors on quality and value for money.

By creating a 'market' in care, the government has distorted the primary tasks of the 'not for profit' care providers. The charities and housing associations now compete openly with each other and with the private sector, substituting the pursuit of power, status and pay by their senior managers for the similar, but rather more frank and honest objectives of the profit-seekers.

The small private care providers

The aims of the smaller private care companies are much less clear. If asked, Reg and Noreen (Chapter 3) would probably define their primary task as something like 'giving care, support and a home to people who have a learning disability and who cannot live independently'. This is a good, straightforward definition of their primary task but it leaves out the need to make a profit. However, with such businesses, making a profit may well be a secondary objective. It may be that a small business is indeed genuinely set up with the prime objective of giving a service and of following a vocation. Noreen was a nurse. She saw the opportunity to run a home and provide residential care in the way she thought it should be done. She needs to make a living from her work; staff have to be paid, and there has to be sufficient surplus to pay for the capital costs of the home; but this is not the same as the profit-making objective of other, bigger businesses. Noreen is in business because of the freedom it gives her to follow her principles of care: principles which she believes would be compromised if she worked for another organisation. This is partly why she so resents and finds it difficult to work with other organisations, such as social services and the inspection unit, which appear to her to be governed by rules and procedures rather than principles. Of course, not all small private providers put care before profit, as she does. Some of the worst cases of abuse have occurred in small Homes which are run solely for profit without a second thought for care when it conflicts with making more money.

The 'not for profit' sector

Although for the 'not for profit' sector (housing associations, charities and local authorities) the primary task should be clear and relatively easy to establish, it is in this sector that it is most unclear. Prior to the 'externalisation' (contracting out local authority services) brought about by competitive tendering, community care and the 'purchaser/provider' split, nearly all local authorities provided their own residential care for most client groups. They were required by statute (the 1948 *National Assistance Act*, Part III, and the 1948 *Children Act*) to make this provision. (This is why the local authority provision was, and sometimes still is, referred to as the 'statutory sector'.) Their primary task, as set down for them in legislation, was to provide 'residential accommodation for persons who by reason of age, infirmity or other circumstances are in need of care and attention which is not otherwise available to them.' (Section 21 (1) of Part III of the *National Assistance Act* (1948)). We must accept that very few local authorities or the managers they employed used the concept of a primary task or knew the words which were the origin of their legally imposed task. Nevertheless, it was to this end that local rates (and, later, community charge and council tax) and the rate support grant were paid to local authorities to make this residential provision. But in the last ten years more and more local authorities have left it to other organisations to provide residential care for them, and they have paid them to do so. Since the advent of community care (when central government social security funding of people in non-local authority residential care was transferred to local authorities to 'purchase' community care), the rush to 'externalise' residential services has become a stampede. 'Not for profit' providers, notably the housing associations, are now 'major players in the market'. This is the sort of language they use. They see themselves in competition with the private profit sector and with each other.

Although housing associations are governed by strict rules of operation, they often appear to act as if they are 'in business'. (Similar transformations have taken place in many social institutions which were established for the mutual benefit of their members/clients but have metamorphosed into quasi-businesses with all the trappings of a commercial company. Building societies are perhaps the most obvious example, where the original idea of membership and mutuality has been superseded by an ethos which is no different from commercial banking.) In hard-headed organisations, like the big housing associations and the major charities, the senior managers find it uncomfortable to be reminded that they should share the objectives which they expect their staff to work towards and that, as managers, their whole reason for existence is to enable the workforce to carry out the primary task. Those who remind them of this are accused of naivety or ignorance. Apart from the occasional publicity stunt and 'photo opportunity' showing them with carefully selected clients, it is unlikely that senior managers will keep themselves in touch with the real business of the organisation.

GETTING AWAY FROM THE PRIMARY TASK

The significance of language

Managers distance themselves in many ways. One is by talking about 'my' staff as if they in some sense owned, or at the very least directly paid, the work-force. A director of social services in a large local authority during the 1970s and 1980s compiled a collection of the circulars and correspondence he sent to the work-force during the many years he managed the department. He published this collection under the title *Letters to My Staff*. He later went on to head a major charity. Such an approach would be more understandable and reasonable in a small care business where the proprietor (owner) is also the manager (as at The Limes), and does personally select and pay the staff. It is her business and the staff work for the manager/owner of that business. Oddly, such proprietors are quite likely to say 'we', 'us' and 'our', rather than 'I', 'me' and 'my'. It is as if they don't need so much to emphasise the proprietorial relationship which they so obviously and legitimately have. Additionally, some may realise that an important element of running a care business well is to include the work-force and to give them some sort of a stake, even if merely notional, in the business. So, for instance, at The Limes Reg and Noreen's care Home business was a 'family' enterprise which included residents and staff in the 'family' culture.

It is common, however, for managers in larger publicly owned organisations (whether or not they are run for profit) to position themselves in a managerial role which they see as distinct and separate and apart from the workforce. Of course, the lofty 'my staff' stance occurs at every level: the head of the Home talks about 'her' staff – or, even worse, 'her girls' (and certainly 'her' residents), but finds that she is owned in a similar way by the service manager, who in turn (like Lok, Chapter 4, p. 33) is 'owned' by the assistant director and the director.

Yet, unlike Reg and Noreen's, this ownership, while being oppressively proprietorial, is far from personal in most of its manifestations.

Since the late 1970s and early 1980s, and coinciding with the political rise of managerialism, managers and politicians have insisted on speaking of the 'delivery' of services – or of its concomitant, 'service delivery'. Indeed, doing anything is described as 'delivering it'. During the same period it has become fashionable to describe cost-cutting reductions in the 'delivery of service' as 'restructuring', 'downsizing' and 're-engineering'. The jargon – which is intended to imply that managers' work is guided by purely rational considerations – is, in fact, indicative of the prevailing attitude which impels managers to cut themselves off from what is really happening to people. The use of evasive language makes it easier for them to erect a buffer between themselves and the real social problems with which clients and workers struggle. They fear that the enormity of these problems may become overwhelming and unmanageable if they allow them to materialise on their desks. 'And anyway', they argue, 'as managers, our own struggles are with the budget, with urgent committee reports, with planning and quality assurance; we just don't have the time to get out and visit the troops.' (Get out of where? What battle is this? And who's the enemy?)

Each year brings more management training and new techniques with which the successful manager must grapple. Managers are promoted and selected on the basis of their technical grasp of 'management', not on how good was the section for which they were last responsible (as judged by the people who used it). Managers seek out particularly high-profile assignments and projects such as 'managing' the 'transfer of undertakings' from one organisation (e.g. a local authority transferring Homes) to another. Negotiating such a 'transfer' (from either side) can be a feather in a manager's cap and will look well on his or her CV. Whether the transfer resulted in a good service and improved care for residents is not seen to be relevant to the management achievement. (It could even be argued that the more catastrophic the results are for the 'service users' and the more disadvantaged the work-force is as a result of fierce negotiation, the more the manager can claim to have pulled off an impressive deal.)

The language in which social care is discussed at academic, managerial and political levels has moved away from and betrays no sense of the difficult dilemmas which workers and clients face together. So problems nearly always seem to be 'addressed'; the word gives an illusion of coolly applied precision but, in effect, 'addressing' in this sense is always distant and often imprecise. Similarly, managers and academics appear to believe that the word 'around', as in 'X organisation delivers services around the issues of substance misuse,' is somehow more exact than a plainer, if not shorter, statement such as, 'We provide X service (specified) to people who have misused drugs.' 'Around' has become widely acceptable professionally to convey the opposite of its real meaning. It would usually be more accurate simply to leave it out. The popular expressions 'around the area of' and 'in the field of' imply that the work might be done without the awkward challenge of engaging with the actual people involved. There is no sense that the worker ever met and worked with a client. What actually happened? What were the results for the client when 'the substance misuse unit addressed the area around harm minimisation'? Did the client know that this is what the worker he met was engaged on? Or were the messy bits of progress and setbacks, the faltering trust built up, and the practical help with the housing department too nebulous to be quantified in the evaluation, even though, if asked, the client might say these were the only real bits of help he ever received. Since the figures produced in the evaluation will be the sole basis for the next year's funding, neither the worker nor the post will be funded in future. The unit's manager will propose a new scheme attracting specific funding for 'skills training' which in turn will be abandoned as new forms of funding for new projects are identified. This manager may go far. He is light on his feet; he constantly raises new funds; he has expanded the organisation, and he keeps abreast of all new developments 'in his field'; but 'on the street' this unit is known for the services it doesn't in fact give, and for the few good workers who have moved on when their particular projects were cut.

New managerialism

Interwoven with and sometimes indistinguishable from what appears to be the managerial ethos of control from above, is a 'new managerialism' in which leadership (an oddly old-fashioned concept) rather than control is emphasised. Many of the 'gurus' of management (such as Charles Handy, John Harvey Jones, Peter Drucker, Warren Bennis, Edgar Schein . . . old uncle Tom Peters and all!) promote what appears to be and can be interpreted and used as a very different management ethos. This is a people-centred management. It is anti-bureaucratic. It is critical of hierarchy, centralisation and systematisation. The proposers of this sort of management demonstrate that it is only when the workforce is truly involved and liberated, and when they also organise themselves well, that real productivity and innovation get going. They show that effectiveness, economy and efficiency (the 'Three Es' of public service management which were hammered home, particularly by the Audit Commission, in the 1980s) can be achieved by organisations who trust and involve their workforce with these objectives. They also explain how the top-down hierarchical organisations cannot achieve the Three Es because they are not sufficiently responsive and because they suppress initiative.

Unfortunately, although many public service managers learn the words of this 'new management', they fail to digest its core messages. So, very often in social care organisations, we end up with a poorly understood combination of the two different management philosophies: control and liberate. We can see the phrases trotted out in 'restructuring' programmes: devolved control of reduced budgets asking fewer people to provide more services. The 'flattening' of hierarchies is driven by the simple expedient of saving money, not by a new ethos of management which gives users of the service and the workforce more control, which in turn will make it more economical, efficient and effective.

Although the messages of 'new management' are fairly straight-forward and are expanded in admirably simple and vivid terms by most of the writers involved, the resistance of public services managers to these messages is remarkable. The tenacity with which they hold on to the old values of distance and control points to an emotional rather than rational resistance. Their readiness to don the costume and speak the lines is nicely parallel to the way in which many men have outwardly adopted the image and persona of 'new men' but still fail to cook the food, look after the children and clean the lavatory. (Of course, these 'new managers' and 'new men' are often the same people!)

THE DESIGN OF A SUITABLE ORGANISATION

Very few organisations start with a blank sheet of paper or a 'green field', and even when they do, planners and managers involved in their design are apt to reproduce a slightly reformed model of organisations in which they have worked or with which they are familiar.

The 'home' element of residential care

On the face of it, it is odd that the organisations which are used for templates of design for running residential services are schools, businesses, voluntary organisations, government (local and national) agencies – and even military models. These are institutional models. Yet the most obvious model of organisation, of which everyone has strong and deep experience, is the least used. Although sometimes people fight shy of using the word 'home' in their descriptions of residential care establishments, there is no doubt that the idea of home is at the heart of the concept of any place designed to provide somewhere to live with other people and to be given care and support. Some of the most influential publications which have set the commonly accepted standards of residential care are quite explicit about the 'home' as a model: *Home Life* (Avebury 1984), *Homes are for Living In* (Department of Health 1989), *A Better Home Life* (Avebury 1996) and *Creating a Home from Home* (Residential Forum 1996).

The management of residential care is distanced and disconnected from running a home or household for many reasons, the most powerful of which are to do with gender and culture. The home organisation, household maintenance and social support at the centre of good residential care are most often associated with women and particularly with 'mothering'. (Of course, men and fathers, often in partnership with women and sometimes on their own or with other men, are also homemakers.) Again, in spite of the political popularity of 'family' and 'home', the skills of creating a good home and thereby, it is supposed, providing the essential, universal social foundations of a good society, are not valued or promoted as ingredients of managing residential care. Generally, therefore, when women become senior managers, most of them act in essentially the same way as do the majority of men in similar positions. The ethos and culture of management are seen as separated and disconnected from creating and maintaining successful homes and households. Those few managers who try to bridge that gap are usually judged to be unbusinesslike and unsuited to their work.

In spite of a mass of 'new management' exhortation to the contrary, most organisations, including those providing residential care, are still designed and controlled from the top down. While that is the case, residents in Homes will continue to bear the burden of a conventional but outdated management which will always let them down because it is obstructive rather than helpful, controlling rather than enabling, and costly rather than economic.

Designing and building an organisation specially suited to residential care

The special sort of management for residential care is one that is created in response to the task. It is modelled on the way the work is well done in residential care, and of how it is well managed within the Home. So we design and build the model from the level at which care is given.

Let us take as our starting point an everyday piece of work between a domestic care worker and a resident. We will go back to the example of The Drive, the Home for adolescents (Part I, Chapter 2), in the year before Bob, the new manager, took over. At the time this was a good, well-organised Home which was clear about its primary task and managed its work to perform that task.

Ellen, the domestic care worker, is a full part of the care team. She takes the lead in matters which are to do with running a therapeutic environment – a household in which attention to the physical state of the Home is seen as intrinsic to the social and emotional support to residents.

This worker understands and promotes the significance of food, the comfort and attractiveness of the rooms and furniture, and the homeliness of bathrooms and toilets. She cleans and cooks but she is not a 'domestic' in the usual sense which largely ignores the importance of the jobs and the relationships developed in doing them, and separates them from the 'professional' care. Other members of staff also clean and cook. Any team member, including the head of Home, would for instance at some time or other take part in the whole range of jobs which the domestic care worker does.

Ellen is helping a resident, Paul, to clean and tidy up his room. Paul is quite depressed and in spite of staff efforts to the contrary, has been staying in bed in the mornings and not going to his work experience placement.

The day before Ellen has arranged to tidy his room with him but he says he has forgotten. She persuaded him to get up and have breakfast this morning and he really seemed to enjoy it, but then he sneaked off back to bed again.

He is lying fully clothed with his shoes on, on top of his unmade bed. By the bed there's an empty can of strong lager with ash and the butt of a hand-rolled cigarette on top of it.

In the last two weeks he has spent a lot of time in his room. Sometimes he goes out at night and occasionally he descends on the company downstairs, is poisonous or simply non-communicative with everyone, takes food from the fridge back to his room, and resists all attempts which staff have been making to engage with him.

Everyone is worried about him. Ellen is one of the older members of staff and her worry about him stays as concern and is expressed as concern, rather than as with some of the younger members of the team, coming out as annoyance and aggravation, and ending in confrontation.

Paul likes Ellen. He doesn't show it but they each know it. She grumbles at him and nags him, and only she could have persuaded him to get out of bed this morning. She cooked him a breakfast she has often cooked for him before. They went through a little ritual which suited him. You could say Ellen spoils Paul, but she has it all worked out.

She is not Paul's key worker but the work she is now doing has all been planned with the key worker and his supervisor. The plan was discussed at the staff meeting so that other team members did not cut across what was being done.

Standing in the room, with Paul lying on the bed studiously ignoring her, Ellen is now gauging her next move. To what extent will she make the room habitable and comfortable? How will she handle the evidence of drinking and smoking? What will she do when she comes across the dog-ends of joints? She has to think of safety, legality and health, but above all she has to think what will help Paul at the moment. She has to communicate both her disapproval and her care and concern, but she is good at that, and there are accepted codes between them. Ellen has the advantage of being old enough to be Paul's granny and not young enough to be his mother or his older sister. She will talk with Paul; she will both scold him and encourage him, without being bright and breezy or pretending that his depression isn't real. He will grunt and complain.

Ellen reckons that she has about twenty minutes before she has to get on with other things. And that will be about all Paul can tolerate too.

She uses the time well. Some tidying gets done, and the room is a bit cleaner. She insists on changing the sheets so Paul has to get off the bed, and she makes him help her – groaning and moaning all the while. She makes him dispose of the can and clean up the cigarette butts. Meanwhile Paul's said something about the work experience and about things at home. He didn't say much in words but Ellen's well 'tuned in' and she's clever enough to have gathered a lot.

She will talk with Paul's key worker about the morning's bit of progress and she will jot a couple of sentences in the notes. But now she's got to get a lot of other practical domestic things organised in the next hour, so she leaves Paul sitting on his bed in a much tidier room, looking through some photographs from two years ago which were found during the tidy-up.

This was twenty minutes' brilliant, skilful, subtle work; but Ellen is working within a carefully designed organisation. Let's look at the organisation surrounding that piece of work (Figure 6.1).

Ellen's work with Paul is within the circle and some of the organisation which is influencing, supporting, guiding and monitoring her work is outside the circle.

During the twenty minutes which Ellen spends with Paul, she is responsible for her work and her decisions; she is accountable to Paul, his key worker, his key worker's supervisor, her own supervisor and the head of Home (who is as yet not part of the diagram).

She is also accountable in other ways to her colleagues, to the duty manager for the day, to the team meeting, to Paul's social worker, and to other residents who may need her attention.

She has many other things to do, so she has to plan her time and work – on each shift, week by week and month by month. But she manages her own work within this context. It is she who manages this intensive twenty minutes, as she will manage all her work that day. Her ability to do the work with Paul is dependent on the extent to which she is managing it.

This is a structure in which Ellen is given the responsibility to take difficult decisions and to work within the boundaries of her demanding job. To enable her to do that she is provided with a structure which

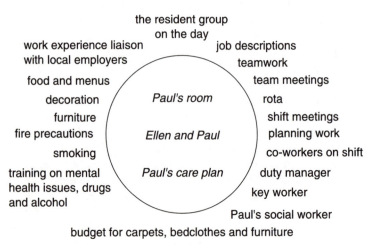

Figure 6.1

gives her support and guidance, access to the necessary information and training, and reliable and consistent staffing – a framework within which she can practise (Figure 6.2).

The structure holds her accountable for her actions. She is part of a complex but clear structure, in which she too has people accountable to her – both as the person taking the lead for domestic arrangements and as a full member of the staff team.

The head of Home would respect the scope and boundaries of Ellen's particular responsibilities; for instance, the head would consult with Ellen before acting on a bright idea for new furniture or kitchen equipment – that is Ellen's sphere of management and the budget for which she takes responsibility.

The head of Home or unit manager's responsibility is the whole Home. Care is the primary task of the Home and everything which goes on within the Home must be managed to carry out the primary task – that is the scope and sum of the unit manager's job.

As with Ellen's work, the unit manager's work exists within the clear boundary of the Home. In order for the unit manager to carry

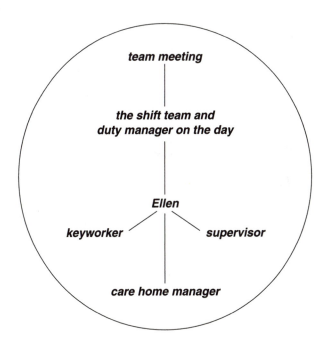

Figure 6.2

out her full responsibilities, to be truly accountable and to have the authority to do the job, outside managers must respect those boundaries. This means that all decisions which impinge on what goes on in the Home (care) and all transactions across the boundary of the Home will be managed by the unit manager or a delegated member of staff (Figure 6.3).

The central manager or service manager should similarly have a clear boundary of responsibility and management, within which she will be responsible for the service itself. That's why she is called the 'service manager'!

This clarity of responsibilities and accountability within defined boundaries for every worker and manager, and for every decision and piece of work, is what all organisations aspire to. Only within The Drive (and only while Sonya was the unit manager) did such clear boundaries become established. In most organisations, clear

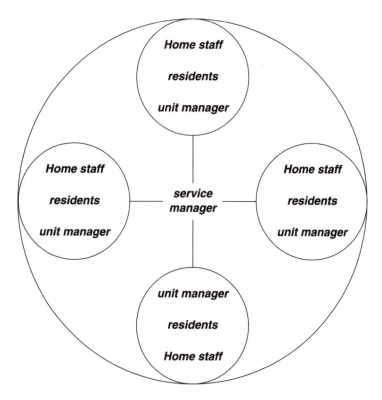

Figure 6.3

management boundaries are an empty aspiration. This is not a bureaucratic exercise whereby senior managers and so-called 'human resources' staff dream up complicated job descriptions, procedures and work instructions. This organisation at The Drive was not designed from the administrative centre; it was designed from the operational centre (the Home) and from the primary task of the centre in action. Unfortunately, this organisational approach did not have much influence beyond the Home. While it works, it is tolerated but sooner or later it will clash with the subverted and distorted primary tasks of the wider organisation, and, as in our story (Chapter 2), it will be destroyed.

Ellen's clarity about what she was doing and what her responsibilities were did not come from the headquarters of her organisation – her knowledge and skills were produced in the Home, through practice, teamwork and supervision. Indeed, it is likely that if managers and administrators outside the Home knew about the extent and sophistication of Ellen's work, they would be very worried by it. They are still likely to be stuck with their limited experience and imagination about what a domestic worker's job should be. This constricted view of management will result two years later in their being able to select and appoint a manager (Bob) who hasn't got a clue about what Ellen does, and who has no inkling of his own management boundaries and responsibilities.

Implementation of the commonly espoused principles of empowerment and job enrichment requires a very different management culture in everyday practice from that which prevails in most organisations.

Although The Drive at that time provided an excellent model of organisation from which the wider organisation of the social services department could have learned and developed, that did not happen. While the immediate manager, the service manager, was persuaded that it really did work and, for a while, found herself managing much better with clearer boundaries, her manager and the rest of the organisation merely felt threatened, anxious and hostile. This resulted, two years later, in the amazing transformation of Ellen from the thoughtful, self-confident and highly competent therapeutic worker illustrated in the example above, to the dissatisfied and angry 'domestic' portrayed in the story in Chapter 2.

Chapter 7

Becoming a good manager in a hostile environment

A manager at any level – Authenticity and commitment – The failure of organisations – The authority to manage – A culture of honest work – The guiding principles for managers – The therapeutic social ecology

A MANAGER AT ANY LEVEL

The job with which a manager is presented in the first few weeks of being appointed often seems impossible. It is during these first weeks that she or he adopts the defences against the anxieties of management with which we are all so familiar – in our own work (if we are sufficiently self-aware and critical) and certainly in observing other managers' work.

Taking responsibility or allocating blame?

One of the first things to understand is that you can't do absolutely everything. Although the popular view is that 'the buck stops here' – that everything taking place below your level is your responsibility – that is not and cannot be the reality. The inaccuracy of such a view and the impossibility of being truly responsible for everything below you become clear if you have done some work on management boundaries (see Chapter 6) – defining what you are responsible for and what other people (both those you manage and those who manage you) are responsible for. So the common, defensive cry of the manager who says, 'I am responsible for everything which you (the subordinate) do, and therefore you may not do anything which is not laid down in procedures,' is reiterated at every level of the organisation. While purporting to define hard lines of accountability, such statements blur responsibility by effectively removing it from every level below the person who is speaking. This rigid way of locating authority within an organisation can logically only mean that the accountability is always at the top – 'The buck stops here'. But when failure or disaster visits such an organisation, blame is the most precisely delineated channel of enquiry, while responsibility and accountability are trampled underfoot in the headlong rush away from blame. Unless there is already a strategy to remove top managers, the finger of blame inevitably points downwards. Huge amounts of the organisation's energy are expended on two questions: Were the procedures in place? If so, who failed to follow them?

Blame

When a residential worker becomes a team leader, and a team leader becomes first a Home manager and then a service manager, it appears that each promotion puts an increased burden of responsibility on the shoulders of the rising manager. In more and more organisations, however, the manager is actually moving steadily further away from the level at which she or he may be precisely blamed for some part of practice going wrong. All the 'manager' must do is to ensure that procedures are carefully written, cover all eventualities, and that she or he at least follows them. It is then a simple, if laborious, task to allocate blame.

The stories in the first part of this book portray managers at all levels trying to find their own ways to manage.

Marcia – not a designated manager but she takes responsibility

In the first story, Marcia took positive steps to move into management responsibilities which were well outside the strict definition of her job. As a responsible, enthusiastic and properly ambitious member of a team, she considered it her responsibility to manage. Had she not managed in the way she did, the weekend at the Una Marson Project would have been a disaster. As it was, it turned into a great success – both for the residents and for Marcia.

Bob – a designated manager who avoids responsibility and blames others

In stark contrast, Bob's pitiful performance (Chapter 2) as a 'designated manager' had deplorable results for residents and staff. However, his approach was possibly more typical of most managers than was Marcia's. He avoided responsibility while adopting all the trappings of a manager. He stayed away from residents and staff; he immersed himself in what he attempted to pass off as essential management paper-work (which included writing new procedures); and he was continually looking for someone (below him in the hierarchy) to blame. As the falsity of his position became more evident to him, he lost authority but he became more authoritarian – and even less effective.

Noreen – who takes responsibility but loses her boundaries

Noreen's position (Chapter 3) was very different from either Marcia's or Bob's. She owned The Limes and had spent years making it a Home, becoming so involved and committed that she could not stand back and analyse the state of the Home or what had been achieved. Nevertheless, she was an instinctively better manager than Bob. Though very ready to tell her staff how to do their jobs when she thought they weren't doing them properly, she would not make them scapegoats. Well practised in and relaxed about giving other people responsibility, she regarded it as her own job to accept responsibility for any faults that were found in her Home. She would defend it and its staff against any criticism whatsoever from 'official' sources, no matter how justified it was. With the recruitment of Thomas as care manager, Noreen was able to re-establish useful boundaries to her role, mostly because Thomas himself was clear about his boundaries.

Lok – who is squeezed between two conflicting approaches to managing

Lok was caught in the difficult position between someone (Rachel) he managed who was prepared to risk taking on all aspects of managing a Home and encouraged other staff to manage, and an organisation of which the upper levels (above Lok) were populated by defensive and controlling managers who were typical of the 'blame downwards' culture so prevalent in large care providers.

Jeeva/Janet – Jeeva enables Janet, his manager, to make changes

Jeeva (the service manager in Janet's story), in a similar position to Lok, becomes the manager who acts as a catalyst in transforming the service. He takes great risks and is supported by a senior manager (Janet) who had become dissatisfied and uncomfortable with the results of her organisation's approach.

Managers make choices between taking on more responsibility or avoiding it and resorting to blame

It is clear from these examples that managers at all levels make choices about how they are going to manage. To put it simply, they must decide whether to take on more responsibility (and, consequently, more risks); or whether to reduce their responsibility and attempt to eliminate risk. Responsibility and risk are avoided by substituting the application of procedures for management and by colluding with a reactive, blaming culture. It is as hard to see the logic or justice of a system that rewards managers for adopting this approach as it is easy to see that it is totally unsuited to managing residential care.

AUTHENTICITY AND COMMITMENT

Knowing yourself

Residential care is an area of work which, as much as any other and more than most, requires the members of its workforce to be themselves. Since 'selves' are never a pure construction of saintly motivations, the members of a staff team always represent a mass of individual and collective contradictions and personal foibles. For the members of a team to pretend to themselves and to other people that their motives are purely altruistic is to refuse to engage with the personal issues. This engagement is essential for effective work with clients. Staff who do not know themselves are unfit to help residents with their own self-development.

Being genuine, acknowledging faults

Although there have been shocking examples of domineering charlatans who have duped, bullied and exploited both residents and colleagues, residents are usually quick to see through a fraud. Staff must be genuine: honestly accept that they have their fair share of ordinary human failings and trust that they can draw on a sufficient stock of the virtues suited to residential work to outweigh these failings. Of course, there are people who go into this type of work for the wrong reasons: for example, principally because they enjoy the power it gives them; or because their main interest in the care-giving relationship is in order to re-enact past wrongs and deprivations; or, in rare but terrible cases, because they are seeking out victims for sexual exploitation. The majority of care workers and managers feel it is too dangerous to acknowledge that most people have elements of the first two in their make-up – and may even have the merest terrifying traces of the third. But not to acknowledge the presence of these traits in ourselves is to block the possibility of working at the deep levels of awareness which will make Homes safer and more genuinely caring.

Marcia – a good mixture of motives

Marcia acknowledged and was open about her main reasons both for doing her current job and for seeking promotion into a management position (Chapter 1, p. 11). Her motivation was mixed; part of it could be seen as self-centred ambition, part as professional development, and a third part as a drive to support and help residents. While she was aware of her motivation, she did not become preoccupied with it; it didn't trouble her. It was a good mixture. (She was yet to face the complications and potential corruptions of being a designated manager.)

Bob – poor motives

Bob, however, is in a very different position. Unlike Marcia, he is a manager now and, if he ever had it, he has lost that good mixture of motivation which drives her. He has taken on the job of head of a Home for children and adolescents because of the pay and status of the job, and because of the car that went with it. His alternative was lower pay as a qualified basic-grade social worker, and although he wanted to get out of residential work, he felt he could not 'afford' to. It was never likely that he would do the job as manager of a residential Home well. He doesn't like the job; he has no good previous experience to bring to it; he has no enthusiasm or professional aspirations for developing the work; he has no commitment to the young people or staff (both of whom he avoids) or to the Home. If it closes and he gets a good deal from being made redundant or 'relocated', that will suit him much better than struggling on with something in which he has no belief.

Commitment and lack of it

Too many managers of residential work, whether managers of Homes or a group of Homes or a service, are in Bob's position. They neither like the work nor do they have any commitment to it. Those who have done the work can't wait to get out of it and those who have not done it, despise or patronise it. Good residential care requires wholehearted commitment from its managers no less than (and, it could be argued, even more than) from its basic-grade staff. If there is no such commitment from managers and staff, residential care is always a failure for the people who use it.

Every new manager will be examined and tested by residents and staff. This test will be more searching than the selection and appointment process. The team members whom Bob joined as manager had established their commitment to the primary task, and it would have been difficult for Bob to convince them of his own commitment – even if he had had it. But he 'ducked out'; he withdrew. He never even tried to do the job. To the residents and the staff he was clearly a fraud.

Organisations which use and abuse staff

It was not only Bob who lacked commitment and authenticity; his managers and the organisation he worked for were uncommitted. Residential care was an expensive burden on the department. In their view, children's Homes should be closed so that cheaper and less troublesome alternatives could be found. Although they may not have been aware of their underlying motivation for appointing Bob, they had chosen well, because the last sort of person they wanted to manage a Home they were considering closing would be someone like his predecessor, Sonya. She had a total commitment to the work, did it well and was of continuing use to the organisation only in so far as she could 'sort out' those Homes which they could not close. The senior managers of the department therefore exploited both Bob and Sonya: one, bribed by money and a new car, for his convenient ineptitude which would make the closure of his Home easier, and the other, attracted by the challenge of managing a difficult Home, for her rare ability to commit all her energy and talent to making it work well, even though they would close it as soon as they could.

THE FAILURE OF ORGANISATIONS

The declared purpose of organisations is to support the work you are doing, yet, by lacking a core commitment to the primary task, organisations are more of a threat and hindrance than a help. You become a manager within an overarching organisation. Its culture and attitudes will always be with you. Even though it is a well-kept secret which, as a member of a social care profession, one is expected to keep well hidden, it is true to say that most organisations which run residential care do not have a fundamental belief in it – whatever their 'mission statements' may declare.

The big care companies

In Chapter 6, we saw how the larger private companies will put their profit and their shareholders first. (In doing so they may sometimes manage to provide excellent services – at a price.) They would be quick to diversify if they saw better profits elsewhere or experienced drastically falling profits in residential care.

The 'not for profit' sector

Many public and 'not for profit' organisations have been more than willing to get out of residential care. The large children's charities, having made their names and collected much of their money on the basis of looking after children and young people in Homes, closed establishments almost as quickly as the local authorities did throughout the 1980s and 1990s. They are now open about their reluctance to re-establish children's Homes (Sparks 1997). (In 1978 one South London local authority ran about fifty children's Homes; less than twenty years later they had none, and were placing children in poorly supervised Homes and foster families miles outside the borough.)

The motivation and 'bad conscience' of some charities

The National Children's Home (now NCH Action for Children), the Church of England Children's Society (now the Children's Society), Dr Barnado's Homes (now Barnados) and the Catholic Children's Society accommodated thousands of children in their Homes (and some were 'exporting' children to Canada and Australia until the late 1960s (Humphreys 1994)) but now they have only very few residential Homes to manage. Many of the 'not for profit' organisations, by turning their hands to campaigning on behalf of children in residential care and to contracting 'new' non-residential services with local authorities, have attempted to dissociate themselves from a long history of poor management and abusive services. (The fact that many Homes within these large charities succeeded in providing a 'good enough' experience for children, in spite of the appalling management record, is a tribute to the strength of belief and the will to survive of residents, staff and some heads of Homes.)

A dispiriting context

The charities, the big private care companies and the powerful housing associations which are taking over the care of adult residents have no better a record than the old mass providers of children's Homes. Within such a dispiriting context, it is only where there are uncompromising commitments from individual managers (at all levels), and the genuine involvement of staff and residents that residential care can be a good experience.

The economic and policy pressures

There are many interconnected reasons for the decline in the provision of residential care for children and the rise in the number of Homes for adults. The foremost reasons are financial. The law and government public policy and financing led to the closure of the local authority and voluntary children's Homes and encouraged the opening of many private children's Homes (among them many small, unregulated but highly profitable Homes). Local authority accommodation for adults (including older people) and long-stay hospitals were closed and – using financial inducements – the government encouraged the proliferation of private and voluntary residential Homes in their place. The local authorities and voluntary organisations which used to run nearly all the children's Homes were pleased to abandon residential care because for many years they had failed in their management of it. Similarly, while many of the local authorities wept crocodile tears, they were relieved to close, sell off and lease out their Homes for adults because of their shameful inability to run them well. Local authorities were stuck with agreements on pay and conditions for staff which made their own provision much more expensive than the 'independent' sector (see Chapters 9 and 11). They were only too willing to make contracts for care with organisations which employed staff on abysmal wages and conditions which the local authorities would not be able to inflict on their own staff.

There are exceptions to this distressing picture, but they are far fewer than a careful reading of brochures, annual reports and policy statements would have us believe. Realistically, this is the generally depressing context which confronts the new manager of residential care. Regrettably, many new managers will capitulate in the face of the power of these organisations. In doing so they will deceive themselves; they will perpetuate institutional abuse and neglect, and betray those people for whom they work – the residents.

THE AUTHORITY TO MANAGE

The word 'authority' and words linked with it are used in many different ways: local authority and health authority, management authority, to give and to have authority, to bear authority and to exude authority, to be authoritarian, to be authoritative, to gain authority, to wield authority, to exert authority, to authorise (payment or action). While there are usages which at first sight appear to be neutral (local or health authority), and others which point to an inner sense of authority (to be authoritative), these words are generally used to assert that one individual (or group) is in a position to 'command and control' others.

The sense of authority

For managers of residential care it is the sense of authority – an inner, personal, quality – that is such a vital ingredient for doing the job. While 'command and control' authority will undermine and block the capacity of the manager of a Home to establish therapeutic communication (see p. 18) in a supportive environment, the inner quality of authority will be the channel through which much of this communication can flow.

Where does this sense of authority come from?

Managers have real authority when they are clear about their task and role, and have belief in themselves and others, and in the ethical and intellectual basis of the place or service which they manage; but they will have achieved this quality of authority only through questioning, doubting and wrestling with each fundamental issue of their work. Nor will they have reached once-and-for-all conclusions; there will still be doubt and a continuing quest for further understanding. They will have learned from a combination of example, experience, teaching, supervision and reflection. They did not become fully fledged authoritative managers overnight. Their authority waxed and waned, and waxed again. Some of their authority was given to them by people who recognised it in them or passed it on to them. It is an inner quality which is evident to other people. The expression of this sort of authority and its recognition are mutual; they form a connection, a relationship, between people.

Parental authority

Images of parental authority are useful in drawing out the distinction between these two kinds of authority. Parental authority is also very relevant to residential care. A mother or father expresses love and care for a child through holding and feeding, through guidance and support, through encouraging the child to become the person she is; certainly, through setting boundaries, but also through helping the child to set her own boundaries – to have, as she grows up, her own sense of right and wrong.

The negative effects of 'command and control'

Managers lacking inner authority resort to 'command and control'. This is the external authority which the manager with inner authority has tested, questioned and challenged. It is the authority which an authorita-tive manager shuns. Authority which wields power, which manipulates, threatens and takes over, is utterly unsuited to residential care. It is the authority which most users of residential care have experienced as harsh, unhelpful and unfeeling. Contact with it is bruising and belittling; it is reminiscent of so many other situations in which residents have found themselves to be powerless – as children and as adults. In the face of such authority, residents become merely compliant or angry and unreasonable; they are apt to lose their own authority, to lose their voice, to find themselves alone and deserted. This authority dresses itself up in power – power over people. It brooks no emergence of people's power to make their own changes and advances. It is often male and White; managers display its power in suits and cars, in ownership. They are well paid and unlikely to live in the area in which they work. They manage for other people services they never imagine they will use for themselves. This authority associates only with other 'authorities'. These authoritarian managers talk finance, contracts and tenders; they work at desks and are brought coffee by people without authority. They invent and reinvent – and reinvent again – their own jobs, their own management language and their own tasks. This authority maintains itself in power, while all below it lose theirs. It is constantly on the look-out for new members of its élite: the bosses. Often it deals with opposition by incorporation; union bosses and people who campaigned with the powerless find themselves being invited to associate with those whom they previously opposed, and very soon they too become fully fledged members, even if they belong to a different branch. This power authority always looks above itself for advancement and below itself for recruitment. It takes 'hard' decisions in the 'real' world. In this version of the language, 'hard' means that other people's services and jobs are sacrificed, and the 'real' world means their construct of the society which provides them with a highly paid job but in which they do not live or participate.

The status of residential care

Residential care has a low status, lower even than the declining status of nursing. It is low-paid work; it is staffed by an undertrained and poorly developed work-force; a much higher than average proportion of workers are female and Black; the hours are long and 'unsocial'; and the work itself is seen to be demeaning (often described in some sectors as 'shovelling shit'). But most significant of all, the users of residential care are the defining factor in its low status. They are the embarrassing, the expensive and the expendable. Those who look after them are caricatured as saints, as lazy, low-grade spongers, or as abusers and exploiters. Readers may find it uncomfortable to face the reality which underlies society's terrible neglect of residential care and its resentment about paying for decent services to vulnerable people. These feelings are usually kept hidden. They surface only when a scandal unleashes the revulsion, rejection and anger which the general population feel against those who have to be 'in a Home' and against those who work 'in a Home'.

Contradictory public attitudes

Our capacity to sentimentalise and 'care' about those who live in residential Homes, and, in almost the same breath, to revile and rail against them, is universal. The exploited and neglected child whose parents mistreated him and who was rejected and deprived by residential care workers, only needed the love and commitment which readers of the newspaper reports feel they would have been prepared to give him. Yet that same child becomes a 'little thug', a 'rat' or 'evil' when the same newspaper recounts his string of apparently motiveless and heartless crimes; readers will be baying for his blood and his permanent incarceration under a bread and water regime. A teenager who would gain massive public sympathy for the emotional, physical and cultural impoverishment of his early childhood, is widely condemned as 'safari boy' if a visit to Africa is proposed as part of his rehabilitation and treatment. The idea that a daughter could 'put' her mother into a Home and that staff in the Home could then mistreat the old lady who was always so gentle and 'wouldn't hurt a fly' appals the reader (who would, of course, never reject his own parent and for whom the mistreatment of such an 'old dear' is revolting). But the same reader loves the jokes about 'gaga geriatrics' in Homes, about Zimmers, false teeth, elderly 'sex maniacs' and incontinence.

Residential workers have to struggle with these awful contradictions within themselves, and with the effects of such extreme attitudes on the public – their neighbours, workmates and families. Residential workers who declare that they 'love' children, old people, or people with learning disabilities are also capable of hating them. An apparently pure motivation for their involvement with caring for such people is likely to cover, or defend against, an element of repressed hatred.

Managers' opportunities to dissociate themselves

Managers of residential work have more scope and opportunity for dissociating themselves from the object which fuels these passionate fantasies of care and punishment, love and hate. Like the detached newspaper reader, by avoiding the direct challenge of the client, a manager is free to condone, collude and condemn with impunity.

Challenging the defences of the organisation

The manager's authority to manage has at its core the manager's own principles, and all good managers will at some time find themselves in conflict with their organisations.

All social care organisations tend to arrange their operations in ways which protect and promote the well-being of the organisation and its managers while reducing the real service to their users. The organisation learns and changes only through constant challenge to its way of operating. People who use the service will challenge by their very presence and their demands; basic-grade staff will challenge because they will find their jobs more difficult to do precisely because of the defences which each organisation builds to protect itself; but whether managers will challenge their organisation (and thereby improve it) will depend on their commitment to principles and the primary task. Each manager will be tested and will have to ask herself or himself the questions, 'To whom am I primarily accountable, my organisation or my clients?' and 'In this situation, will I stand up for my principles and beliefs, or will I do as I am told?' Of course, this is why it is dangerous (for organisations) for a manager to be too close to the clients and the primary task. If you do not know the clients of your service and you see yourself as just one of many managers in a large organisation of which you are a conscientious employee, and you take it as axiomatic that the organisation always has the best interests of the client at heart, you do as you are told. This way you will join those social workers and managers who parted children from their families and sent them to Canada and Australia where many were abused (Humphreys 1994), who ignored and later covered up abuse in Homes for people with learning disabilities, and who found ways to silence or get rid of staff who blew the whistle on bad practice in Homes for older people. You will join those managers of social services in North Wales who ignored, denied and stifled the desperate cries for help coming from staff and residents in their foul institutions for children during twenty years of sustained abuse.

Hard choices

As a manager you have hard choices to make. The material rewards of becoming a procedures person (both writing them and following them), and of being discreet and subscribing to the organisational view, will be high. If you do conform in this way, it will be at the cost of your professional and personal integrity, and as a manager of residential care you will eventually be found out. However, it may not matter to you either that you will lose your professional authority with residents and staff or that you will be ineffective as a manager of a Home, because you may have your eye on 'higher' things for which your conformity will recommend you.

If you choose the alternative path which takes you close to residents and basic-grade staff and to all the dangers and risks which they face, you will become a 'difficult' manager and you are less likely to prosper in either your own organisation or in any other.

Fortunately some organisations and their most senior managers welcome and support 'difficult' managers. People's integrity is respected and dissent, risk-taking and creativity are not only tolerated but actively encouraged, much as they need to be within any residential

Home. Residents, staff and 'difficult' managers become the agents of change and development; application to achieving the primary task becomes the key factor in all decision-making, and the organisation becomes truly authoritative and learns how to run residential care services.

A CULTURE OF HONEST WORK

A dishonest culture

Bob (Chapter 2) had the misfortune to be tutored in management by being deputy to Clive, a corrupt, lazy bully. In spite of the increased regulation of residential care, there is much that goes on which should not. There is still widespread petty fraud – the fiddling of money, timesheets, supplies, provisions, time off and sickness, rotas, telephone calls, stationery, photocopying, travel claims – as of course there is in most organisations. While this dishonesty is tackled only in the conventional ways – by 'tightening up', by increasing surveillance and control, by disciplining those who are 'caught' – the special significance of dishonesty in social care and particularly in residential care is missed. A pernicious culture is left untouched. Much valuable time is spent policing staff in homes, and much more is spent by the same staff inventing ways of evading detection or substituting new ruses for ones that have been rumbled. Not only is this effort wasted, it has a negative effect on staff who shift the responsibility for their own probity (so vital to their direct work with residents) on to their managers. This is made even worse when they know that their managers, like them, are up to every 'scam' available. Dishonesty becomes a subcultural game: get away with whatever you can without being caught. There are many instances of residential care managers being persuaded to resign (and even sometimes receiving substantial financial inducements to do so) when their dishonesty has been found out. Such events are usually well known to staff and residents, and, in work with young people, hopes of helping residents to resist or reduce delinquency are destroyed.

Small dishonesties are punished; major ones are concealed

It's no good giving a domestic worker a written warning about arriving at work ten minutes late but not showing it on her timesheet if you, as her manager, take an extra day off at the weekend and claim that you are sick. It's no good disciplining the head of a Home for making personal international phone calls at the expense of the council if, during the next winter, you, as the service manager, steal the council's time to watch cricket in the Caribbean sun! In Bob's case, both his manager and the director of his department appeared more committed to running their lucrative private business than to getting on with the jobs with which they had been entrusted. So Bob, without strong principles of his own and lacking a clear commitment to the work to guide him, found the prevailing organisational culture difficult to resist. His dishonesty was more subtle, but nevertheless it was still a betrayal of trust – the trust which both residents and staff should be able to put in a manager. In some organisations it is more likely that a kitchen assistant who steals a loaf of bread will be dismissed, than will a senior manager who sets up an elaborate operation using council staff, premises and equipment to steal, store and resell thousands of pounds' worth of food which a major retailer regularly donates for residents' consumption. (As with all examples used in this book, these are all real. The manager in this instance received a very favourable retirement 'package'.)

Misplaced attempts to enforce honesty and 'standards' without tackling the dishonest organisational culture

In spite of painstaking attempts to define and proceduralise ethical practice in organisations, there is a growing discrepancy between the standards of honesty which the public (including service users) have a right to expect from social care organisations and the standards which many managers practise. This is in part a result of the current political and moral climate of competitiveness and individualism in which self-advancement and avarice are regarded as desirable attributes. Managers who are caught up in this culture lack the maturity and inner authority to establish boundaries for themselves but rely on their organisations to define what is right and wrong for them. In such a culture everything is fair game if there is no rule which forbids it. Instead of using their own principles to know what staffing levels are required to give adequate care to residents, many managers take their staffing levels from their local inspection unit, and simply see how few staff they will be allowed to get away with. These are the same managers who will readily make rules for other people on the basis that employees too are immaturely dependent on external rules for regulating their personal and professional behaviour at work. Regarded from this perspective, it becomes easy to see how such organisational cultures are totally unfitted to the proper conduct of residential care. 'Homes' cannot be homely, mutuality cannot survive, and trust cannot grow under such regimes. Most obviously in work with children and young people, managers who invent rules for residents, but clearly have few moral inhibitions themselves, and who manipulate and evade those rules which the organisation sets out for them, are not to be trusted. All managers set an example; many set a very bad one. It should not surprise us that some young people who are 'looked after' by such organisations become distrustful and delinquent.

THE GUIDING PRINCIPLES FOR MANAGERS

In the first part of this chapter we have considered how easily it all goes wrong for the manager. We have seen that your suitability to manage residential care will be determined by the extent to which you:

are willing to accept your responsibility and be primarily accountable to residents;
demonstrate commitment and authenticity;
question, challenge and participate in changing the organisation;
have a sense of authority;
and whether you are intrinsically honest.

With these determinations and qualities as your foundations for taking on this difficult job, there are two fundamental principles with which to practise. You must:

engage and *respond*;
seek to *promote* and *sustain* the processes of *growth* and *learning* by which a Home becomes a *'therapeutic social ecology'*.

Only by treating the Home as a holistic, integrated entity can you avoid the common and destructive modes of managing: defend and react; isolate and intervene.

Are these principles just good sense and experience expressed in highfalutin language?

On one level the guiding principles of doing and managing the work can be seen as instinctual and straightforward common sense. Like having children and bringing them up, it is assumed that most women know how to do it. They don't have to be told, to read books, or to go on courses. Even some men can bring up children without additional tuition. Although they may not themselves have been brought up to do it

– their mothers never showed them how to change a nappy – they can use their own good experience of being looked after, to look after others. The skill of caring seems as if it is innate, but with a little further examination it will be seen to be something which was learned through good experience and becomes in part instinctual because such experience has such profound, unconscious effects.

And again like bringing up children, managing residential care is full of honest mistakes, pitfalls, contradictions, and finding yourself doing and saying things which, within seconds, you regret. It is the balance itself that is crucial. What we are talking about here, as with the raising of children (Winnicott 1964), is 'good enough' management. Even if there were such a state as perfect management, it would not be desirable, because it would rule out the constructive process of learning from the consequences of the manager's honest mistakes! Good management is therefore always imperfect.

Some very successful residential Homes have been run using the abundant supply of good sense and experience which is shared amongst the staff and managers. It is only comparatively recently that the absence of comprehensive procedures and of management expertise in residential work have been regarded as serious flaws in the service. There is now less specific training for the work at diploma or qualifying certificate level than there has been for forty years. After a succession of scandals and subsequent inquiries, politicians and policy makers have created a large and complex system of training, inspection, and managerial and administrative processes which were proclaimed and justified as initiatives to transform a service. Ten or more years later, the service as a whole is little changed. However, there is a huge army of trainers, consultants, managers, administrators and inspectors whose job it was to change things during this period, but who have failed in that job and yet are still employed at salaries far outstripping those of the people who actually do the work. Nor do the members of this élite group know much about residential work; most of them have never done much of it, and their training and expertise is in other areas (not least in selling themselves and their services). It seems odd that we should so easily accept this situation, but again it is a comment on the low status of residential Homes and their residents. Most of us would be nervous of travelling on an aircraft piloted by someone whose training and previous experience had been in driving a lorry. Yet even experienced residential workers often fail to trust their own judgement and skills, choosing to take instructions from people who have little relevant knowledge and experience but an abundance of conceit.

Professional development on the job

The most valuable and lasting professional development in residential care has at its core good work experience with staff who have high principles and standards in a Home which provides excellent care. Staff are trained to notice a situation, to assess it, and to respond – all within seconds. For many years The Limes (Noreen's Home, Chapter 3) was just such a Home. Noreen and her two colleagues established very good practice within a homely atmosphere. Care assistants learned the job and became excellent practitioners. When Thomas (the new care manager) was recruited, The Limes had reached the stage where it required his professional approach to be added to (not to replace) the apparently more instinctive and common-sense methods of Noreen and her colleagues. The Home was nearly destroyed by the overbearing intervention of inspectors and the detached, misdirected requirements of regulations. Had it not been for the good sense of the chief inspector and his ability to recognise the genuine quality of the place, the residents of The Limes might well have lost their Home, and an invaluable and rare training resource for staff would have disappeared.

The 'Law of the Situation' (i.e. 'Engage and Respond')

At The Limes the principles came from within. Unknowingly, Noreen and her colleagues used Mary Parker Follett's 'Law of the Situation' (Fox and Urwick 1973) to manage their small organisation. The concept of this 'law' is that each situation, when analysed, has its own logic: its history, its context, its present state and its own development or solution. It is the situation itself which provides the way forward and gives its 'orders'. A mechanic investigating a malfunctioning piece of machinery analyses the situation and takes steps to repair it. A cook preparing a meal for a dozen people takes her 'orders' from the situation; she analyses all the complex factors involved – time, place, availability of ingredients, the likes and dislikes of the diners, costs, equipment, presentation, her own particular skills, the rewards and risks inherent in trying out something new, her previous experience of this group of people, and countless other factors which all spring from the situation. In Chapter 6 (p. 56) we saw how Ellen, the domestic care worker at The Drive, managed her work by a similar process. She 'responded' in accordance with the dictates of the situation with which she had 'engaged'. Although Parker Follett was writing about industrial and commercial business management, her 'Law of the Situation' is equally applicable to managing residential care. She explains that one of the overriding advantages of this 'law' is that it means no one has to take orders from or to give orders to anyone else. The situation itself provides both the 'orders' and the authority to carry them out. The management function is to visualise and to comprehend the whole context of which this situation is part, and to coordinate and integrate the work-force and other resources, thus enabling the individual worker or each small team to get on with their jobs, and together to set the organisation to its task. This 'management' function applies at all levels; it does not have neat cut-off points below which workers do not 'manage' but simply take their orders from the situation – they do both. As we saw in the example of Ellen's work (p. 58), while she applied herself to the situation and took minute-by-minute decisions, she too had to visualise and comprehend the whole situation of which she was part.

Like many helpful theoretical conceptions, the Law of the Situation can seem a little trite. Because she conforms to it and thinks it comes naturally, Noreen would say, 'Well, that's what anyone with an ounce of common sense would do!' But it is not what most residential care managers do, and the higher up the hierarchy they get, the less likely they are to do it. They will dress up their observation and analysis in all sorts of quasi-scientific management jargon and they will issue orders. Even if they include staff in making decisions, it will not be because they believe the decisions belong to the staff and that residential Homes can work well only when people (including residents of course) can take their own decisions. No, they will justify this comparatively rare policy of staff involvement by calling it 'delegation' (foisting their difficult decision-making on people who are lower in the hierarchy) or 'empowerment' (a charitable process to make managers feel good, which is halted as soon as it gets serious and threatens to change anything).

The Law of the Situation is an active and practical concept. While not excluding assessment, planning and reviewing – the necessary activities supporting action – it puts responding to events and taking action at the very centre of all management. For those people who use a service – in this case the residents – such a principle of management is of great benefit. The Law of the Situation dictates that a manager takes steps to improve a poor service immediately, as well as considering the long-term implications and changes required to prevent the fault being repeated.

The Law of the Situation (Engage and Respond) as applied to a dirty lavatory

At a most basic level, a manager of a Home for older people, walking into a dirty lavatory which is dangerously unhygienic and where the floor is wet and slippery, must do something about it immediately even if that entails cleaning it himself. He will 'engage' with the problem with a mop and bucket! He has a duty to ensure that no resident of the Home is put at risk by using that lavatory. The situation dictates that he must take action ('respond') in the short term, but in taking action in the short term, he will also uncover the longer-term laws of that situation by asking such questions as:

How long was the room in that state?
How often and how is it checked?
Do other staff use this lavatory and, if not, wouldn't it be a good idea if they did?
Would all staff see it as their job to take action immediately?
How come I, the manager, am the person who is aware of this problem?
Have there been accidents (falls) in this and other lavatories?
Is there a problem with one particular resident?
Where are the cleaning things kept?
Are they sufficient and suitable for the job?
Does the present state of this and other lavatories encourage cleanliness?

Because the manager took quick action himself, the situation not only posed these questions, but the manager concentrated the power of the situation, and stimulated much sharper and more focused attention from staff.

The discovery of a dirty lavatory by the manager should lead to (a) the immediate cleaning of the lavatory; and (b) (if it was not an isolated and very unusual situation) action to prevent further similar situations. In obeying the Law of the Situation at these two levels, the manager and the staff team will come across other situations which will give further 'orders'. (For example, in discovering where the cleaning equipment is kept and what chemicals are used for cleaning, the manager may go on to check whether the manual of hazardous substances is up to date.) What is not needed by residents, but what often happens, is that the organisation reacts by surveying, analysing, reporting, and proposing convoluted impractical remedies. Managers and staff get drawn into protracted negotiations about keeping lavatories clean, monitoring systems, job descriptions, standards, etc.; meanwhile, the lavatories stay dirty and residents are put at very great risk – to their health, safety and dignity.

It is this dynamic interaction – engaging and responding – between unfolding situations and using them to make progress, between real events and real responses, which makes the Law of the Situation (and our residential care version: Engaging and Responding) such a complementary partner to the principle of Sustaining the Therapeutic Ecology.

THE THERAPEUTIC SOCIAL ECOLOGY

The idea of a therapeutic ecology has its roots in social learning theory (Jones 1979), group psychodynamics and the experience of therapeutic communities: people learn from their own experience with each other, and absolutely everything which goes on in the Home is connected with everything else, forming part of the help which people get from living there. Like the Law of the Situation, this is another theory of behaviour which seems obvious once stated – perhaps too obvious to be fully comprehended. Just as we commonly accept that children learn from their experiences of family life – and, less so, from school life – without being deliberately instructed in how to feel, think and behave, so it seems obvious that residents and staff will learn individually and collectively from residential life in a Home. Living and working in a Home will, in themselves and with awareness, reflection and understanding, provide the means of learning about and changing life and work both individually and communally.

Degenerate social ecologies, e.g. prisons

Of course, in too many Homes this living together and learning experience is a negative experience. In these poor Homes the ecology is far from therapeutic; it is polluted and dangerous. The deprivations and punishments of prison and the ideas which underlie the current enthusiasm for sending people to prison are rooted in a crude and negative form of social learning theory. It is proposed that criminals will be 'taught a lesson' not to reoffend simply by being sent to prison; yet contradictorily, the power of social learning is acknowledged by recognising that prisoners will learn to be even more criminal, will learn how to evade detection more effectively in future, and become hardened to moral argument both by their association with other criminals and by the brutalising social 'education' of life in the prison itself.

What is recognised here is that prisoners will indeed learn, and their subsequent behaviour will be influenced, far more by the everyday life they experience in prison than from the isolated 'programmes' of education and training which are provided. On one level it seems rather silly, for instance, to bring trainers and counsellors into prisons to conduct drug rehabilitation programmes with prisoners who are living in a criminal culture dominated by drug use and dealing. While such programmes may have an effect on a very small minority of inmates, on the other more sinister level, the Home Office and prison service use them to hide the fact that the presence of drugs in prisons has been condoned and even, in some ways, promoted at all levels of management. The prison culture – its violence, rape, drug and tobacco use, and its pecking order – is essentially a delinquent agreement between staff, management and inmates, without which, they all tacitly agree, most prisons would be unmanageable.

Prisons are extreme forms of residential institutions, but all 'Homes' are susceptible to similar degeneration – capable of taking on delinquent cultures. In such cultures 'social learning' does take place but not in the form which encourages residents and staff to join together in changing and developing the culture and quality of life as happens in a therapeutic 'ecosystem'.

It is, of course, this positive form of social learning (understanding and sustaining a therapeutic ecology) which can be used as a guiding principle of good management. First managers – at any level – must believe that residential life in Homes can be a positive experience. In other words, they must believe in the value of their work and they must be determined to be part of creating and managing a service of real value to people who use it. Without this belief and commitment (p. 67) from managers, there is little chance of any form of residential care becoming a positive experience. A depressingly high number of managers fail this first test of fitness to manage.

The essential components of a therapeutic ecology

Belief and commitment will make you something of an extremist in most organisations which provide residential care, even in those whose main task it is. You then have to define what it is that your belief and commitment are invested in. What is the principled core of residential work? Definitions abound, but it is your own definition which is vital at this level, not the ones you can take from the books. However, if you believe that residential care should be the best realistic option for all residents (Wagner 1988), your definition will synthesise the special factors in Homes which create a therapeutic ecology.

Clare Winnicott, speaking about residential work with children in 1961 (Winnicott 1971), says that the child living in a Home requires 'something direct and real' – experiences which are completed and which become part of the child's inner psychic reality, correcting the past and creating the future. She says, 'I have made it sound simple, but I know that it is the most difficult and demanding job in the world.' She continues, 'I suggest that the essential skill in residential treatment lies in the worker's ability to *achieve a way of living* [my italics] for a group of individuals. On this basis alone the group can then become an important socialising and therapeutic agency for the individual.' The child – and this applies to people of all ages – is helped by the *whole* experience of residential life, which brings us back to the idea of social learning in a residential community.

What are the special ingredients in this whole experience – the elements of a therapeutic social ecology?

1 Each person will be listened to and communication will be on a person-to-person level, not on 'staff-to-resident' or 'manager-to-worker' level. People have equal rights and status in communication.
2 All aspects of life and work during the whole day and night, from the most individual and mundane to the most public and formal, will be important, and are open to discussion and understanding as significant in the life of the Home, the work of staff and the lives of individuals.
3 Through living their lives and carrying out their work, and through reflecting on, discussing and analysing their own experiences and events, residents and staff will be able and free to learn. Experimentation in pursuit of learning and changing will not be punished when it goes 'wrong'.
4 Authority is personal not institutional. It carries with it personal – individual and group – responsibility. Authority can be challenged and questioned. It is exercised in direct, face-to-face engagement.
5 Staff roles are clear but not compartmentalised. While each member of staff will have her or his own special and specialist experience, skills, interests and knowledge, these are always integral parts of a whole team. Team members, at all levels, involve themselves with the work and life of the whole community or household, and understand that all their work influences and is influenced by everyone else's work. Residents will not, therefore, split and compartmentalise

their needs. This experience of the integrated work team will in itself be of immense help to residents.

6 Residents and workers will have a regular forum (meetings) in which to think about, discuss, learn from and change – and to take part in the management of – the life of the whole Home.

(Hawkins 1989)

(There are several examples in this book of how this framework can be used and each part of it implemented without any grand theory or impractical intellectualising, see, for instance, Chapter 8, pp. 105–10 and Chapter 12, pp. 186–95.)

Residential care is a positive choice (whoever makes it) when residents live a better life in the Home than they would have done out of it. Generally, life in the Home is no less complicated than it is anywhere else, but a Home is inevitably a 'planned environment'; it has to be designed and helped to work – it has to be managed. While we have recognised that many Homes (like The Limes, Chapter 3) are not very deliberately planned and managed, and yet can be pretty good; and others (like The Drive after Bob became manager, Chapter 2), though planned, are very disjointed and poorly managed, creating and maintaining a therapeutic social ecology is usually a hugely complex management task. Successful management of residential care requires more awareness and understanding than direction and instruction; more concentration on group relations and development than slavish adherence to a procedures manual; and more coordination and cooperation than command and control. Like the natural ecology of the environment or an organically managed farm or garden, the social ecology of a Home becomes sustainable and productive when we allow it to function, when we help it to work, and when, using the principles of a therapeutic approach, we apply ourselves consciously to the primary task and protect the Home from anti-task attack and encroachment.

Part III

The practicalities of managing a therapeutic social ecology

Chapter 8

Residents

There was an old woman who lived in a shoe . . .

i Responding to residents' needs
The wide range of urgent needs – Engage or disengage? – Managing risks – People need a home: a good place to live in – The comprehensive listing of needs, rights and values – Putting values into practice – Rights and risks: the dilemmas for staff – Reacting conventionally but irresponsibly to residents' needs – Engaging and responding

ii Power and participation
Participation: window dressing or culture? – Residents participate at The Limes – 'A positive choice'? – Control of finances – Prejudice and discrimination – A cocoon is not for living in – A time of hope

Responding to residents' needs

As we saw in Chapter 6 (Ellen, p. 56), the organisation and management of residential care is best built from the needs of the residents and the staff who are working directly with the residents. 'Grand plans' which start somewhere else – generally at the top, but certainly outside the Home – are usually failures for the people who need care and for those who give it. Many managers will have caught themselves thinking, 'Everything would be fine if it weren't for the residents and staff'! Let us hope that most of them quickly realise that their own jobs depend on 'troublesome' residents, and a somewhat smaller number will also realise that their best staff are likely to be 'troublesome' too (Chapter 10).

In order to create and sustain a therapeutic ecology (Chapter 7) staff must be constantly aware of and responsive to residents' individual and group needs. This is possible only in an organisation which functions as a complex living and learning, adapting and changing organism, rather than as an inflexible machine. Residential Homes are changing all the time. Every time a new resident arrives or one leaves there are important changes. Events and emotions buffet the place around. Residents are deeply affected by other residents. A resident may not have received the phone call she was expecting. An anniversary comes up which no one knows of; or, as sometimes happens, a resident is reminded of an anniversary and may be convinced that it is the day of – say – a close relative's birthday when actually it is not, and staff have no means of knowing what the resident is concerned about. Equally possible is the agitation and upset caused by a persistent memory of a still-born child, or the death of a brother, or some such traumatic event. Without being close and highly sensitive to residents' moods and feelings, staff would have no way of supporting a resident at this sort of time. This organisation (the Home) must be prepared for most eventualities, some of which are predictable but many not.

THE WIDE RANGE OF URGENT NEEDS

In other social work or social care jobs you work with people in short episodes and usually at a distance – on the phone, visiting someone's flat or house, or conducting interviews in the office. Even a whole day at a day care centre is of a different order from residential work. Engagement with clients is relatively limited and protected. You do not usually encounter clients at the most difficult times of their day or night – early in the morning, late at night, in the middle of the night – and of course in other jobs you rarely have to encounter clients when you are half-asleep and have just struggled into your dressing gown.

In other jobs, it would be unusual to be directly involved in the most vulnerable events in people's lives: moments of great loss, getting up and going to bed, arguments with other people, fights, eating, the visit or failure to visit of a relative, incontinence, the onset of Alzheimer's disease, returning drunk or drugged from a party, menstruation, falling and injuring yourself, teasing or threats from other residents, constant extreme pain, the birthday that's been forgotten, granny's death, a nightmare, loss of hearing or sight, paralysis through a stroke, falling in love, sex and sexuality, using the same bathroom as other people, buying clothes, the night before going to court, being bullied at school – the constant exposure of fears and vulnerability.

In other jobs you know these things are happening to your clients; you talk about them; you try to support your clients – but you are not often there with them as the events are happening.

ENGAGE OR DISENGAGE?

The alternatives for the residential team are stark: either the team organises itself and orchestrates its work in a way which enables staff to 'engage' with residents through all these events and to stay with the primary task, or the team organises itself to 'disengage' from these exhausting, frightening and emotionally threatening people (the residents) and the tasks they demand in their support.

Such disengagement is a sort of institutionalisation. It is what most organisations running residential care are adamantly opposed to in principle but unintentionally wedded to in practice.

This tendency to defend against anxiety (Menzies 1970) is always present – in all of us and in all of our workplaces. Organisations both ensure it happens and collude with it – and then occasionally pick off staff who get caught up in it.

MANAGING RISKS

Lok (Chapter 4) was visiting Norwood House following an incident in which a resident had gone out of the Home and was picked up by the police about 5 miles away. Mr Brown lived in the special Alzheimer's unit and went missing on a Wednesday afternoon during the staff meeting. Although there was one member of staff who stayed with residents on the unit, she wasn't aware that he had gone. It wasn't until the other staff returned from the meeting that they noticed Mr Brown's absence. He had lived at Norwood House for only a week. Although he had not shown any signs of 'wandering' during the week, he came with a reputation for 'going missing' from his own home. His son and daughter-in-law were worried about his tendency to go for walks on his own and to get lost.

As soon as the staff had searched the unit for Mr Brown, they informed the duty manager of the whole centre, and she told all staff to look for him on all the units, in the public areas and in the garden. The staff from the unit who were due to go off duty looked around the immediate area of the home, asked in shops and knocked on the doors of neighbouring houses. Meanwhile, as soon as it was realised that he was not in the building, one of the staff from the unit rang the local police to report Mr Brown missing. She also rang his son, who said that he would come straight away.

There was a call at about 7 p.m. from another police station about 5 miles away, to say that an old man answering Mr Brown's description had walked into the police station to ask the way, but wasn't clear about where he wanted to go or where he had come from, nor of his own name and address. He was cold and tired, but seemed unharmed. Mr Brown's son set off to fetch him and the old man was back in the Home having something to eat and drink by about 8 p.m. He said that he had been going home but had got lost.

Initial enquiries by the duty manager established that the care worker who had stayed with the unit during the staff meeting had had to spend about ten minutes with one of the residents in her bedroom helping her to change, and then had been distracted by another resident. Although there was a well-established practice on the unit, whereby the staff constantly kept an eye on the twelve residents and regularly 'counted' them mentally, there had been about twenty minutes before the end of the meeting when the worker had not been able to make this discreet check. It was almost certain that Mr Brown had simply walked down the back stairs and out of a ground floor exit during that time.

The staff team on the unit were well experienced and had extensive training in caring for people who had Alzheimer's disease and other forms of dementia. A lot of their time was spent doing things with and talking with residents, rather than merely trying to keep up with their physical care needs. By being constantly alert to residents who wanted attention or who were feeling like taking a stroll around, they had reduced the problem of 'wandering'. Even so, Mr Brown was not the first who had gone missing. Six months previously, one of the residents had several times left the building without being noticed. On one occasion she had ended up in hospital after being knocked down by a car when crossing the road.

The unit was not particularly well designed for residents with dementia. It was on an upper floor of the building and there was no area where people could take a stroll and be physically active without disturbing others. The staff had proposed that the unit should be moved to the ground floor, that a large conservatory should be added, and that part of the garden should be fenced off and made private for the unit. This would enable residents to use the conservatory and garden whenever they wished to without being able to wander out of sight. Naturally, there were arguments against these proposals – not least, disrupting the residents who had to move and finding the money for extensive work on a building that had only recently been expensively converted to its present use.

The relatives of the woman who was knocked down by the car were naturally very upset about the incident, and although they thought very highly of the Home, they felt that there must be some way of staff preventing a recurrence. 'We know you can't lock them in but isn't there something you can do?'

At the team leader's suggestion a small and inexpensive battery-operated alarm was installed on the fire exit door at the top of the stairs which the resident had used when wandering off. This had exactly the desired effect. The sound of the alarm reminded her where she was and what she was doing whenever she opened the door, whereupon she immediately closed it and returned to the sitting room. And staff (who, of course, hurried to the scene when they heard the alarm) gained an increased awareness of her pattern of activity and, consequently, an increasing ability to anticipate her needs.

It was a simple solution to one very worrying problem, but it posed others. Another resident was in the habit of opening the fire exit door and going down the stairs to look out of the landing window and gaze at the garden. She did this a dozen times a day; and because she never wandered off but always returned safely to the unit, staff had no reason to dissuade her from this pleasurable activity. But now, of course, the alarm went off each time she opened the door. Although she simply ignored its piercing shriek, other residents were very disturbed by it, and staff were wasting precious time investigating repeated 'false alarms'. It soon became only too evident that the quality of life in the unit was being impaired by these frequent disruptions.

Clearly, the alarm was now doing more harm than good. It had served its purpose. The resident for whose safety it had been installed had soon got the message. Within a fortnight her wandering had ceased to be a problem – partly because of the alarm, but chiefly because she had become much happier and more settled as staff had learned to understand and respond to her particular needs. It now seemed most unlikely that she would wander again. For this very good reason, and after much discussion, staff decided to switch off the alarm. (Six months later, when the assistant director was looking for scapegoats after Mr Brown had wandered off, the team on the unit would be severely censured for taking that decision.)

As 'service manager' Lok was kept fairly well informed by Rachel, the manager of Norwood House, and by other staff at the Home, with whom he often spoke. He had been well aware of the difficulties the unit was grappling with (including 'wandering'), and he had admired their flexible, thoughtful and practical responses to them. They were typical of the approach that Rachel encouraged and supported. She was always reluctant to tell teams what they 'must' do; she expected them – and very willingly helped them – to find their own answers. Through a similarly supportive and trusting relationship with Rachel, Lok also played his part in enabling staff to make their own decisions and in fostering a learning organisation which was able to respond quickly to residents' needs. (It is important to note that residents themselves were encouraged to do their own learning and take their own decisions.) Lok had a very different relationship with some of the other establishments in his group. When faced with almost any problem, it was the managers of these homes who would ring him for directions.

Similar incidents of 'wandering' had taken place in another Home, one of which led to a substantial out-of-court settlement with angry relatives. After that the local authority's insurers had threatened to increase their premiums unless the organisation was able to demonstrate that it had taken measures which would prevent its residents from wandering off the premises. In response to this threat an elaborate and expensive alarm and video system was installed. This satisfied the insurers; and it gave the authority great satisfaction because it enabled them (with the agreement of the inspection unit) to reduce the number of night staff in the Home from three to two. That staffing reduction paid for the surveillance system in one year; but the quality of life and care in the Home deteriorated even further. It was now common practice for the two night staff on duty to spend much of their time in the office watching the monitoring screens. Surveillance – not care – had become their prime concern.

Ruefully, Lok wondered how long it would be before the staff too were 'managed' by some similar method of surveillance. He was ashamed of this imposed, wrong-headed, technological solution, which had admittedly stopped any further occurrences of wandering but had also reduced the staff role from active, involved, responsive caring to mere security and the provision of physical attention. It was not his own solution. It was produced by the local authority's safety officers in conjunction with a surveyor from the buildings and maintenance department who had recently read an article on new security systems in a trade journal. They regarded this first scheme as a pilot project. Then, later, they had put a joint proposal to the assistant director (Lok's manager) to install similar systems in all the homes. As the safety officer argued, in the six months since the installation of this system there had been no further incidents of residents put at risk through wandering, and in the previous six months there had been ten in that one home. The figures spoke for themselves; and the borough's insurers (having paid out once already) were keen as well.

The assistant director had circulated all the Homes with instructions to cooperate with the companies which would be making preliminary surveys in order to tender for the major contract to install the systems. He also spelled out the 'self-financing' aspect of the system (the saving on staff costs), and assured the Homes' managers that the deal on staff reductions was currently being negotiated with the unions. The inspection unit had already indicated that an extension of the pilot project was acceptable to them.

When Rachel received this circular, she was furious. She immediately wrote back to the assistant director telling him that she would certainly not cooperate, and setting out all the reasons why, in her view, the proposal was absurd and abusive. She was all the more angry because of the work which all the staff at Norwood House were doing to find the proper way to handle this. This was their own work. This was what residential work was all about: thinking, responding, adapting, and meeting individual and group needs; not waiting for some ignorant and detached outsiders to solve problems by remote control.

She felt let down by Lok, whom she expected to protect her from this sort of nonsense – because he usually did. She just managed not to voice her strong suspicion that there was something crooked going on: that some of the officials involved (perhaps even the assistant director himself) had a personal or financial interest in this contract. She didn't trust any of them, didn't want anything to do with them, but was always ready to fight if they came trampling over her work.

The assistant director was fed up with Rachel's attitude. They (Norwood House) had let another resident (Mr Brown) wander out of the building and get lost. In his view it was particularly irresponsible that the resident had 'absconded' (his word) during a time when they insisted on having all the staff on duty (the staff meeting). They were lucky he hadn't been killed; and the assistant director was now determined that Rachel and her dangerously independently minded staff would come into line. Her letter alone was grounds for taking disciplinary action against her; but before going down that road, he intended to force Lok (or 'Luke' as he called him) to show which side he was on. Lok was caught in between. He knew that Rachel was doing her job properly and needed his support. Norwood House was a place where the needs of the residents shaped the care work and its management. That was obviously how it should be. But Lok also knew that if he, like Rachel, was seen to be ignoring or countermanding orders from the most senior managers, his own job would be at risk, and Rachel and the whole of Norwood House would then be exposed and vulnerable to the destructive and oppressive urges of senior management.

PEOPLE NEED A HOME – A GOOD TO PLACE TO LIVE IN

Broadly speaking, residential care is intended to look after (care for) and to accommodate people. For all but very short-term residents the residential Home becomes a person's actual home during the time she or he lives there, and, for some – like young people moving into independent accommodation – for a period after leaving. So, for all residents who are appropriately placed, the Home is intended to meet the complex mix of needs which people's own homes usually meet. This mix is physical, social, emotional, intellectual, cultural and familiar – indeed familial. Noreen (Chapter 3, p. 21) describes The Limes in its early days as 'like one big family'. Professionals are properly wary of such a description but – when it is true – it does encapsulate what many clients want from a residential Home, and what, therefore, would largely meet their needs. The dangers of such a description are that: (a) it may sentimentalise and disguise the institutional aspects of the Home; (b) some clients (particularly children and young people who have been abused in families) certainly do not want or need anywhere which might turn out to be like their own family; and (c) the 'family' concept creates a dependency and intimacy which intrudes on the independence of people who want to do most of their living on their own but also need twenty-four hour care. In the last case, we might question whether such clients would not prefer to be accommodated in a form of sheltered housing (having their own flats) where such care is immediately available.

THE COMPREHENSIVE LISTING OF NEEDS, RIGHTS AND VALUES

The rights and needs of residents are usually expressed in the – by now well-known – list below:

- fulfilment
- dignity
- autonomy
- individuality
- esteem
- quality of experience
- emotional needs
- risk and choice

This list, first set out in *Home Life* (Avebury 1984) is important and was certainly useful when first compiled. Subsequent publications have varied and refined the list, e.g. privacy, dignity, independence, choice, rights, fulfilment (Department of Health 1989 *Homes are for Living In*).

The problem with such lists is that they become repeated mantras which everyone is expected to know off by heart, which are used as the format for inspections, and which become part of the conventional wisdom of residential care. These ideas initially stirred up and invigorated the work but have now been allowed to sink to the bottom and become mere pious sediment. As with William Blake's 'Jerusalem', inspirational words which were once written to question and challenge institutions have been incorporated into the litany of institutional power. The principles on which residents might have once campaigned and established their own rights and power, are smugly reflected back at them from glossy statements held up to deflect criticism and demonstrate the institution's comprehensive credentials. The three-page chart in *Homes are for Living In*, which sets out the six basic values of residential care (above) and lists the areas (below) in which an inspector (or a manager) could examine the implementation of these values, is a brilliantly comprehensive and concise exposition. It asks the inspector to examine the following areas against each of the principles below:

- physical environment
- care practices
- staff
- staff training and development
- procedures

- case records
- documents
- meals and mealtimes

Managers or inspectors using this chart should in theory be able to assess and review the implementation of the commonly adopted principles. So why don't they? All the managers and the inspection unit involved with the decision to install video surveillance equipment in the local authority Homes (of which Norwood House was one – see the example on p. 95) subscribed to these principles and yet were able to break most of them. Even government guidelines which attempt to protect the rights and choices of residents fall into disuse when managers' other priorities intervene. With the rise in fostering and the use of private Homes for children and young people, clients are being sent to live far away from their home areas to placements which have been inadequately checked and monitored (Hume 1997). This is in contravention of the guidance from the 1989 *Children Act* and flouts all standards of good practice.

Once managers stop listening to residents (and their friends, relatives and advocates) and to staff, they become immune to their needs and demands. Once they commandeer the principles, they throttle them by entangling them in their procedures and proclaiming them as their own. Thinking – in its reflective, creative and critical senses – about the principles and their application to the work stops. The principles die and are embalmed. They are memorialised in – often rather worn and tatty – corporate statements of purpose and standards, and 'customer service guarantees' which are found pinned up in offices and entrance halls, and which are passed, forgotten and unread, dozens of times every day.

PUTTING VALUES INTO PRACTICE

The accepted values of residential care are embodied in the description of residents' entitlements set out and defined in *Homes are for Living In*:

Privacy: the right of individuals to be left alone or undisturbed and free from intrusion or public attention into their affairs

Dignity: recognition of the intrinsic value of people regardless of circumstances by respecting their uniqueness and their personal needs; treating with respect

Independence: opportunities to act and think without reference to another person, including a willingness to incur a degree of calculated risk

Choice: opportunity to select independently from a range of options
Rights: the maintenance of entitlements associated with citizenship
Fulfilment: the realization of personal aspirations and abilities in all aspects of daily life.

Although it can never be easy – perhaps it is never possible – to ensure that residents receive all their entitlements in full, managers who are genuinely committed to the values of residential care will strive to achieve that ideal outcome.

Norwood House provides a striking example of a Home in which residents' entitlements were the first priority. Both Rachel (the manager) and the staff were genuinely committed to putting the values of residential care into practice. Consequently, they were alert and responsive to residents' individual and group needs; and they encouraged residents to participate in running the Home by consulting with them when making decisions. Together, they – manager, staff and residents – were making Norwood House 'a good place to live in'.

Rachel reacted angrily to the assistant director's circular (p. 95) because she knew that the surveillance system he was proposing to install would severely impair, if not destroy, the privacy and independence (amongst other rights) that residents at Norwood House now enjoyed – and to which they were entitled. She didn't need to be reminded that it was her duty to try to minimise the risks of 'wandering'; but – unlike the assistant director – she was not prepared to tolerate the Home being turned into some kind of 'secure unit'. She always encouraged staff to think about the problem and supported their attempts to find realistic but principled ways of dealing with it. Both Rachel and her colleagues were well aware that by pursuing this policy they were incurring 'a degree of calculated risk'; but, as our next example shows, they were willing to accept this. It was the price they readily paid to avoid damaging the quality of life of other residents while trying to protect a 'wanderer'.

RIGHTS AND RISKS: THE DILEMMAS FOR STAFF

Mr Brown, the resident who got lost after walking out of the Home, was known to like going for walks on his own, but he had 'gone missing' from his own home and his son and daughter-in-law told the staff at Norwood House of this tendency. To have someone keeping an eye on you all the time is intrusive and an invasion of privacy. As citizens, people are free to come and go as they please, and not to be watched. Set against those principles is the 'duty of care' which can be expected from staff in a residential Home.

The staff's initial plan with Mr Brown was to observe this 'wandering' behaviour and to keep an eye on him, but only to the extent that they would any other resident. Since 'wandering' was not initially unusual in several residents on the unit, the staff had developed the habit of constantly making a quick mental count of residents and being particularly alert to some residents' absences. As in work with other client groups – especially children – the staff at Norwood House developed a 'sixth sense' which alerted them when something might be wrong. Experienced staff sense the total atmosphere of a group living unit. The 'feel' of the unit is mainly composed of all the things which residents bring to it, and the absence of a resident changes the 'feel'. This was not only important for 'wandering' but for other risky situations which some residents might get into. The practice on the unit was to be very attentive to changes of mood, and to get involved with residents, sometimes to divert them from unsuitable activities or, for instance, to take a short walk with them if that's what they seemed to be most keen on doing. The team tried to balance the residents' rights and freedom to do what they liked with their own duty and obligation to protect them from un-warranted risks. Current methods of working with each resident, hour-by-hour changes and developments, concerns and risks were recorded in each resident's notes and briefly discussed at each hand-over meeting (three times a day), and notes were made on progress.

Mr Brown had settled well in his first week and had shown no inclination to wander off anywhere. The staff meeting that week had been a team meeting which took place on the unit. In his second week, however, a full staff meeting at which all the teams were present (except one worker from each unit) took place in the large common room on the ground floor. Most of the residents on Mr Brown's unit were untroubled by this; they were used to it. But it was assumed (after the event) that what was to him the unusual absence of all the staff, except one, disturbed him, especially when the one remaining member of the team was also not to be seen anywhere for about ten minutes because she was helping another resident to get changed in her bedroom. Mr Brown particularly valued the company of the women on the staff and liked to sit and talk. He had also discovered some small ways in which he could lend a hand, for instance tidying the books and cleaning the glass in the fire doors – which he insisted on doing with newspaper and vinegar.

It was thought later that, on the afternoon of the staff meeting, he had been looking for the staff, had been perplexed not to find them, and had simply looked further afield by going through the fire exit at the top of the stairs, where previously a temporary alarm had been fitted to alert staff to the wandering habit of another resident. He continued down the stairs, found the outside exit at ground floor level and went into the garden; then, forgetting his original mission, Mr Brown began to walk 'home'.

If the alarm on the fire exit door at the top of the stairs had not been switched off, the member of staff on duty in the unit would have been alerted to Mr Brown's departure at once; but it had indeed been switched off – and for good reasons (see p. 93). As for the video surveillance system which the assistant director proposed to install in all the Homes, that would flout every principle which the staff at Norwood House had worked so hard to uphold. In spite of the very real limitations imposed on residents by their disabilities and mental and physical frailties, staff constantly thought about how they could support them in enhancing their privacy and dignity, in maintaining independence, in making choices, in exercising their rights, and in finding fulfilment in their lives at Norwood House. Mr Brown's 'wandering' was a problem for the staff team to think through – and to which, because they had a good grasp of the values of residential care, they would find a solution that was sensitive to his and other residents' needs.

On reflection, the team agreed that leaving one worker on the unit during the staff meeting did not adequately meet the needs of the residents (especially with the additional needs of Mr Brown). The worker herself was not at fault – it wasn't as if she hadn't attended to residents' needs as fully as she could – but, even after helping the resident to get changed, her attention was taken up by the urgent needs of another resident, and she hadn't noticed that Mr Brown had gone. If she had done the quick count (which they were all in the habit of making) just then, she could have got someone from the meeting, and he might not have wandered much further than the garden. This was of course all in hindsight. The worker was inclined to blame herself, but her colleagues knew that simply leaving the problem with 'what might have been' and allowing her to take the blame would get in the way of a proper thinking-through of the situation. Each of them knew that they had done exactly the same thing many times.

REACTING CONVENTIONALLY BUT IRRESPONSIBLY TO RESIDENTS' NEEDS

At this point the team on Mr Brown's unit at Norwood House could have done what many staff teams do. They could have 'disengaged and defended'. Such a reaction takes many forms:

refer it 'up' for a manager to deal with ('You can't expect us to look after so many people and come to the staff meeting too; you decide what we should do')
blame the resident ('We can't cope with Mr Brown as well as all the others; he shouldn't have been admitted');
blame the building and equipment ('There should be alarms and videos');
ask for procedures and risk assessments which will 'decide' what to do in each instance, so staff simply follow the procedure ('Give us a rule to follow');
blame the organisation ('They should provide and then this would never have happened').

ENGAGING AND RESPONDING

However, the staff team were operating in a culture (a management culture) of 'engaging and responding': Mr Brown's care was their responsibility and they were all very concerned about him and also about discharging their responsibility to him and his family, and for the unit.

The directive from the assistant director about installing the surveillance equipment was an incomprehensible insult to their professionalism and commitment. It would be like offering an established creative artist a 'paint by numbers' canvas for her next picture. In the other Homes, the staff had jumped at the chance of relinquishing this central part of their work: reflecting on problems, understanding them, thinking them through and creating principled ways of responding.

This is why it is essential that the people who are doing the work fully participate in the decision to accept (admit) residents (see Chapter 6, pp. 59–61). When a professional team of workers take on a new client, they are committing themselves to working with that client. To make this decision, they must be fully informed of the resident's history and circumstances, and they must have a plan to work to (care plan). But if a team has not made this decision, they cannot commit themselves to the resident or to the plan. They will not take responsibility to engage and respond; instead, as soon as something goes wrong (as with Mr Brown), they will simply withdraw – disengage – and defend. Organisations are then left in the position of having to substitute directives, procedures, disciplinary codes and technological solutions in place of responsible, skilled, committed social care. With such inadequate and wholly inappropriate substitutes, they simply cannot do the job.

Power and participation

The first part of this chapter has been about managing residential care in response to residents' needs. The second part is about residents' power and their participation in management. Of course, participating in decision-making about how your own care is provided and about matters which affect the whole Home is very much part of residents' ordinary human needs, whatever age they are and whatever disability or frailty they may have. It is very common to hear staff (and even residents) dismissing the possibility of such participation on the specious grounds that residents are physically, intellectually or emotionally impaired and cannot, therefore, attain what is supposed to be some 'normal' level of functioning. When you hear such comments, you can be sure that staff are also considered (and, tragically, may consider themselves) unfit to take part in the management of the Home and of their own work.

PARTICIPATION: WINDOW DRESSING OR CULTURE?

The genuine participation of residents in managing a Home always takes place within a broad continuum. It is characterised by the attitude and culture created by staff, residents and the organisation within which the home exists. If 'participation' can be found only in the regular convening of residents' committees, in suggestion boxes and complaints procedures, genuine participation is unlikely to exist at all. All Homes should be very wary of mistaking the formal trappings of 'democracy' for a real, messy living democracy. As in so many other areas of managing residential care, we must be suspicious of the gloss and we must look for the substance – and know how to recognise it when we see it.

The way in which Marcia (Chapter 1) encouraged participation and drew residents into the management of life at the Una Marson Project will have not gone unnoticed by most readers. However, the formal trappings of participation at the project, such as the residents' meeting, were not very convincing. The substance was in what individual staff actually did. Marcia knew that she could not work effectively for and with the residents without participation, but she, like residents, had little confidence in the formalities or in the commitment of managers.

Bob (Chapter 2) was, of course, quickly destroying the culture of shared responsibility which had been built up at The Drive over the several years that Sonya was manager there. Noreen (Chapter 3) had always scornfully answered the questions on her pre-inspection questionnaire about participation with 'no' or 'not applicable', leading any inspector who didn't know The Limes to conclude that there was no participation by residents, and that Noreen did not consider people with learning disabilities capable of taking part in this way. That was not the case. Noreen hated the very idea that the sort of give-and-take, the arguments and agreements, and the 'family' culture established in her Home would be categorised as 'participative'. From reading inspection reports, she knew that a highly institutional neighbouring Home was described by inspectors as 'participative' simply because it had formal monthly residents' meetings at which residents were 'consulted' . When asked by the inspector on a previous inspection how the decision was taken for a group of residents and staff to go to Tunisia for an autumn holiday, Noreen said bluntly that she herself had decided, and that since the residents weren't paying for it, it wasn't much to do with them. This was a provocative and mischievous distortion of the truth, but Noreen was aware that exactly that attitude had prevailed in the other Home and yet the inspectors had been told that such decisions were taken by residents at their meetings. Thomas (the new care manager) would be able to develop aspects of the highly participative informal culture that Noreen and her colleagues had established at The Limes, formalise them where necessary, and in addition communicate them to outsiders in an accurate way (see p. 25).

Lok (Chapter 4) recognised that Norwood House had developed a strongly participative culture of management and life, but that this was threatened by the hierarchical bureaucracy of the local authority. Finally, Janet (Chapter 5) saw that the hopes for future development of the care services lay in Jeeva's talent for working with people at every level (which he did with what appeared to be instinctive ease) and in his capacity to give people (or to let them take) responsibility, so that both residents and staff blossomed in such a remarkable way in the group of Homes which he managed.

Our examples demonstrate some of the wide range of possibilities for resident participation and its links with management. We will now examine more closely how Thomas built on the informal culture at The Limes.

RESIDENTS PARTICIPATE AT THE LIMES

When Thomas arrived at The Limes as the new care manager he knew he was coming to a good Home run by honest and principled people. What they had been looking for was a manager who could both maintain and cherish the homely, informal 'family' atmosphere and yet develop a professional and formal structure. To Noreen, the Home's joint owner and previous care manager, this seemed an impossible task; but to Thomas, who had the benefit of professional care and management training to add to his good experience and creativity, this combination was required in any good Home. In some ways the first steps towards formalising participation and decision-making had been taken in the way Thomas was recruited and selected. For this job it wasn't going to be good enough to rely solely on the old common-sense and intuition approach. Drawing up the person specification, setting out the method and criteria by which the successful candidate would be selected, and – most of all – involving the residents in the selection all took planning and a lot of thought. Thomas was immensely impressed with the fact that residents participated in a very real and practical way – something which he had often thought about himself and had heard a lot of talk about, but had never known really to work.

At first Thomas simply observed how some very effective informal communication took place between everyone – residents and staff. To begin with, he built on what existed. There were handovers of a sort between shifts of staff but, through his own regular attendance, Thomas encouraged a more structured and reliable method. He asked that each resident was considered and reported on. He got people to make brief notes. Next he set up a weekly staff meeting. At this meeting also, he insisted that the work with each resident was discussed before talking about the business of organising the Home; and the meeting ended with a half-hour training session. While the staff began to enjoy this new organisation of meeting, talking and decision-making, and learned to develop the meetings themselves, Thomas was also working on the residents' communication. In any case, the residents were very interested in the way in which the staff had begun to meet and talk, and would often join them in meetings after individual residents had been discussed, so a model and the beginnings of a new culture were starting to grow.

Thomas noticed that residents were meeting regularly but no one referred to the gatherings as meetings. After the evening meal, which staff and residents ate all together in the large dining room, discussions would often develop. Staff sometimes initiated them by taking the opportunity to announce some important information – anything from an impending inspection, to an outing, or to someone's birthday. Or they would simply announce that they were going to be doing something interesting that evening or at the weekend and ask who would like to come along or take part. But also questions were asked: problems and proposals about organising life together in the Home were put to the assembled company by residents or workers, or sometimes both. Sometimes it would be a complaint or a dispute which was brought up, talked through and, usually, settled. By sitting with residents at mealtimes and eating with them, staff encouraged talk. Even though a few of the residents were unable to hold a conversation they were nevertheless included in other people's talk. Residents found this was a way of raising concerns. They would enlist the support of the worker sitting at their table with them, and then they had the option of the issue being put to the whole company either directly by themselves or through the member of staff (or not at all if that's what they wished).

Some of the residents were not sufficiently coherent to make themselves understood and relied on the advocacy of staff; others might sometimes stay for only a part of these discussions before losing the sense that what was being debated was important to them and their lives in the Home. But by first making the staff more aware of the significance of these gatherings, and then by helping many of them to discover that they were highly skilled in encouraging residents to communicate and participate, Thomas coaxed the post-meal gathering into becoming just a little more of a formal event.

As they were when he arrived, Thomas reckoned that these 'meetings' were better than anything he had experienced so far in any other Home, but after about six months' very careful work, the meetings developed even further. Thomas talked about the full participation of residents and staff in the management of the home both inside the meetings and at other times. He put the idea around and got people talking more about it.

One of the issues at The Limes, as at any other Home, was that the residents (and indeed the staff) had very different levels of capability

– particularly in thinking and communication. After all, The Limes was a Home for people with learning disabilities, which were usually combined with some other circumstance making the residents unsuited or unwilling to live in their own separate accommodation. Outsiders (and most of the people who are in the work and should know better) find it difficult to understand or envisage how people with very limited intellectual capacity can participate in the complex business of running a Home. The same is thought of children, people with mental health problems or with physical disabilities, and of very elderly people. Of course the underlying prejudice which, in common – and even professional – opinion, excludes them from this partici- pation is not so much to do with the realities of their reasons for needing to live in residential care, as with the fact that they do live in care and should, therefore, according to this mistaken opinion, be passive receivers of care, not the active organisers and directors of their own lives and Homes. Thomas did not think like that. Nor was it the long-established culture of The Limes, for Noreen had never thought like that and most of the staff had enthusiastically adopted her approach.

Thomas considered that everyone living at The Limes had intel- lectual abilities. They were all able to make important decisions of some sort and to participate in group decision-making in some way. While only a few of the residents could read and write, and only some could speak fluently, all of them had ways of expressing their likes and dislikes, and of communicating complex thoughts and feelings to the people who had learned to communicate with them.

As Thomas 'floated' the ideas about making shared decision- making more full and formal, the debate became heated and passionate. People were very anxious about losing the 'naturalness' of the established way of doing things and feared the pressures of anything more formal. He found himself in a small minority amongst staff and residents. He talked a lot with Noreen – and with Reg, who would often surprise Thomas by his sensible grasp of the principles of residential care. After the inspection, Noreen was more and more able to stand back and not to interfere. She had tremendous confidence in Thomas and – almost daily – recognised in his steady and gentle but challenging and far-sighted leadership that the future of The Limes was exciting. At first she found the idea of full and formal participation strange. All her old prejudices about the dead hands of bureaucracy and procedure told her that 'formalising' things would spoil them. But she also perceived Thomas's commitment to maintaining the homely, informal and family spirit of the Home, and she found herself persuaded by his arguments. Thomas was doing with Noreen what he was doing with everyone else: he was not asking her permission; he was not trying to get her on his side; he was talking about his ideas, testing them out, getting her view, her ideas; he was thinking with her and stimulating further thought.

Thomas knew also that, without being in any way devious about it, he was achieving the very state of participation which he was hoping was attainable. At a formal staff meeting discussion, he got agreement to propose a special meal to follow the staff meeting on the next Thursday evening. He would put this to residents at the post-meal gathering. He said that he wanted a regular occasion when the important decisions affecting everyone in the Home could formally be taken together. He proposed that they all (including all staff) should have a special meal each week (maybe a buffet) and that after the meal they should have a formal meeting (chaired and minuted by members in rotation). All the big decisions should be discussed at the meeting and if there was disagreement some things could be decided by a vote. Residents' families, advocates and friends would be welcome if specifically invited by residents themselves, but would not be able to vote. If a vote ever came down to a split between staff and residents, staff would not be able to out-vote residents simply by dint of being in the majority.

Thomas proposed that the first meeting would be held on the next Thursday. There was a good discussion. Some staff repeated the arguments – some in favour of the proposal, but more against it – which they had put forward in the staff meeting. Staff sat with residents who needed support and sometimes, making it quite clear that they were doing so, they spoke for residents who could not express to the full gathering the views they were indicating to staff sitting with them. Some residents and staff were concerned about the extra cost of a special meal and whether the food budget could stretch to it. When the arguments had been heard and everyone who wished to had made their points, Thomas said that he thought the meeting was discussing two proposals: the first was whether to have a weekly special meal on a Thursday evening; and the second was whether to set up a formal weekly household or community meeting to take place after the special meal. The proposals were then voted on and the first was unanimously agreed; the second was narrowly defeated, with more or less equal numbers of residents and workers voting together each way.

The first special meal was a great success and there was the usual informal discussion afterwards. At the third Thursday meal Thomas wanted to discuss some major spending options with the residents. He had already outlined the issues at the staff meeting in the morning but all the staff had felt that the decision would best be made with all the residents. The choice was between an extension with a conservatory to make more communal space, and a new bus to replace the ten-year-old one which was becoming unreliable. These two possibilities had been much discussed and thought about already, and everyone had a real interest in both, but whichever was chosen would rule out the other for at least another two years.

Thomas raised the issue and briefly put some arguments for and against each proposal, but said that at the moment he didn't know which he thought was the priority. Some residents joined in, and then one, Ann, who enjoyed debates like this and always spoke up, said, 'Why don't we decide with a vote, like we did before?' One of the staff said, 'Yes, that's a good idea, Ann, and why don't you chair the discussion and take the vote at the end?' Without further pursuasion, Ann changed places with someone who was sitting in a large upright armchair at a table at one end of the room. She banged on the table and asked for order and said, 'OK, I'm in charge of this meeting. Who wants to say something? Put up your hand and I'll call you.' Ann chaired the meeting with a wonderfully economic directness. She was alert, fair and encouraging but she was also strict about sticking to the point and not wasting time. She loved doing it and in subsequent months turned out to be the most regularly elected chairperson, although many other people – staff and residents – took their turn when elected.

The meetings became established but they never turned into the formal and bureaucratic quagmire which those who had initially opposed them had feared. Occasionally, when there was nothing for the meeting and no one wanted to raise anything, the meeting would end within two or three minutes.

Thomas had got what he had hoped for, but he had done so without manipulation or trickery. When they turned down his original proposal, residents (and staff) had themselves taken initiative and power, which they later used to set up their own meetings when the time was right to do so. Thomas was delighted and thought that they had done it as well as they possibly could. While Thomas remained a very powerful and influential person and no one ever doubted his fitness and capacity to be the manager, they now perceived his power and their own in a very different way. He could be opposed and he would accept it; they could take charge and yet he retained – even increased – his authority.

Although they did not fully understand what had happened or how it had happened, the inspectors were very impressed with this development. At least they recognised that the sort of participation that had been achieved at The Limes was very different from the 'participation' – of which Noreen was so scornful – that they had found in the neighbouring Home.

The story of how residents' participation was nurtured at The Limes illustrates the real and practical possibilities. Homes for all client groups can aim for a similarly high degree of involvement by residents in management; but – as the example shows – the staff, and particularly the manager, must manage such involvement if it is to be achieved.

'A POSITIVE CHOICE'?

By dint of coming to live in a Home, residents will always be in a vulnerable, dependent and relatively powerless situation unless, as at The Limes, managers and staff take positive and carefully thought-out measures to enable them to participate in decision-making. In spite of the universally proclaimed (but rarely practised) principle that people make 'a positive choice' to live in a Home, the vast majority of residents of all ages have not themselves made any such choice. They have not been able to do so. It is usually other people – family, courts, doctors, social workers, community care managers – who collaborate to make decisions about admission to residential care. In the general view, residential care is the 'last resort': people are 'put in a Home' rather than choosing to go and live in one. Furthermore, when policy-makers talk of 'care in the community' they – and indeed the general public – wrongly assume that residential Homes are not included in 'the community', in spite of the fact that the finance with which local authorities fund adult placements in residential care is 'community care' money. Of course, if the alternatives are – as they used to be – a massive institution or a small 'group Home' then the latter is considered to be more 'in the community' than the former, but, in the view of all but a very few, residential care remains a very poor alternative to living in your own home. Consequently, the minority of residents who have genuinely chosen to live in a Home rather than in their own accommodation or with their families are regarded as having made an odd choice.

Prejudice against residential care is reinforced by widespread disapproval of those like-minded people (usually young) who choose to live together in a large mixed household, finding this a satisfying and convivial way of life. Disparagingly categorised in the tabloid press as a 'commune', such a household is generally regarded as being a refuge for 'deviants' who choose to live in squalor, to indulge in drugs and depravity, and whose disturbing attitude to authority threatens 'the fabric of society'. Fed by lurid stories of 'what goes on in these places', fantasies of social breakdown and moral dissolution run riot. This – so the argument goes – is what happens when people are allowed to set up a self-governing community in which they attempt to sort out their own lives in their own way.

The false and silly assumption that self-government necessarily leads to disorder and what is popularly described as 'anarchy' is prevalent in social services departments and, all too often, is shared by the managers and staff of residential care Homes. They see themselves as being in charge of residents who have to live in Homes because, for various reasons, they are judged to be incapable of living a 'normal' life in their own homes. Believing that 'such people' would behave irresponsibly if they were given any real say in how their lives are run, most managers oppose all radical measures which would enable residents to have real power, opting instead to control them. Though rarely admitted, and frequently disguised by policy statements to the contrary, it is generally accepted that such control must be exerted to protect residents from their own physical, mental or moral shortcomings.

Where the perceived threat of 'anarchy' is most frightening – as in Homes for children and young people – managers usually try to maintain order by inventing a system of rules and controls. Although these are always resented – and often resisted to the point of open rebellion – they are regarded by most managers and staff (and by the general public) as being essential. How else, it is asked, can young residents, many of whom are 'delinquent', be prevented from making trouble? In most of these Homes, management policy is based on the belief that if their residents are encouraged and supported in running their own lives, they will inevitably and quickly 'get out of hand'. (Yet, of course, all guidance to good practice and ordinary common sense tells us that 'learning to run your own life' is central to becoming a responsible 'grown-up'.) And, though well concealed, control is generally the first priority for the managers of Homes for adults (such as pensioners and people with learning or other disabilities) where there is little likelihood of an outbreak of violent disorder. It is a different form of control –

insidious rather than openly coercive – but it is no less damaging to residents' dignity and independence. The older residents are, the more readily they may accept rules and regulations imposed on them 'for their own good' – thus acquiescing in a management policy designed to keep them in a state of dependency by denying them their entitlement to participate in decision-making.

In Homes where staff collude with these deep prejudices and anxieties, residents become victims of a regime which offers them little opportunity of finding real fulfilment (Department of Health 1989 *Homes are for Living In*). In others where staff confront and challenge entrenched opinions and attitudes – in themselves, in their organisation, in society at large – residents will be able to do the same. But to confront and challenge is not easy. It is neither easy to combat prejudices nor safe to pursue policies that run counter to them; but when staff are genuinely committed to putting the values of residential care into practice they are ready to battle with difficulties and accept risks. Noreen did it without much thought but with plenty of principle and passion. Thomas did it in a planned and thoughtful way, which then enabled Ann (the resident who first chaired the meeting) and other residents to recognise their right and to establish their power to control their own lives.

CONTROL OF FINANCES

Some inspection units are now stopping private providers (especially smaller businesses) from administering residents' income (usually benefits and pensions); but too many organisations running residential care continue to take control of residents' finances, including the personal spending element which is still persistently referred to as 'pocket money'. It is obvious to anyone who values their own independence that it is quite wrong to hand over the control of your income to the person or organisation from whom you buy your accommodation (and all that goes with it) and your (very expensive) care services. Would you entrust your pension book or your salary cheque to your landlord? If, for some reason, you could not administer your own finances, you would find (or be helped to find) someone close to you and well known to you, or a volunteer, or a completely independent professional to act on your behalf (see Chapter 11, p. 172).

Children and young people under the age of 18 have the same need and – according to their age and level of maturity – the same right to control their own money. It is not proper for staff to use children's money to control them, any more than it would be right to use the provision or deprivation of food to control them – or anyone else, for that matter. The underlying principle here is that it must be clear to residents (and to staff) that their money is their own. In some circumstances – if, say, residents are using their money recklessly or illegally (for instance, to buy drugs) – staff have a duty to try to protect them from misusing their own property; but at no time should residents' money be 'confiscated' or be subject to 'fines' imposed by the Home as part of its attempts to control.

Culturally, money is a source of power. Even a little money enables people to make decisions about spending (or saving) it. Although children may need help with using and enjoying this power, learning how to handle money – to budget, to save and spend it – is essential to taking increasing control of your life as you grow up. Through living in a participative Home, children and young people can have the additional opportunity to learn how to manage money from the experience of being involved in decisions about the communal budget.

PREJUDICE AND DISCRIMINATION

We have seen how simply by being resident in a Home, people are often regarded as abjectly dependent, in need of surveillance and control, incapable of decision-making, and unable to take reponsibility for their own lives and finances. In combination with these oppressive views, residents have to contend with the more general prejudices and discrimination which prevail in the wider society. The attacks on their survival and their sense of well-being inherent in the negative experience of residential care are compounded by this widespread preconception from outsiders of what it is to be a 'resident'. ('Inmate' is a word which often emerges when outsiders are searching for a description of this powerless, dependent being.)

A much higher number of women than men live in Homes for older people and a similarly high proportion of women work in nearly all types of residential care. Although it should not be the case, while the rich often can afford to stay at home and pay for services to be brought to them, poorer people who need the same level of service, but are not directly paying for their own care, are provided with the cheaper option of residential care. So a higher proportion of poorer people are living in Homes. Prejudices about age and disability follow people into Homes and can become doubly oppressive. Homosexuality is hardly acknowledged in Homes (in spite of pious policy statements to the contrary); so gay and lesbian residents are isolated and cut off from the sources of strength and companionship which they may have built outside the Home in resistance to prejudice and attack. Racism is manifest in different ways in respect of different client groups. In most Homes for older people a Black resident is likely to be one of a very small and visible minority. She is likely to encounter considerable prejudice from other residents even if a majority of staff are Black. However, the staff are rarely encouraged to use their different backgrounds and experience to contribute to the Home's resources. Apart from occasional and very artificial 'multicultural' evenings, when curried goat and rice and peas suddenly become the main meal but aren't seen on the menu for another six months, there is neither any sign that the Home values the cultural diversity of its staff team or existing residents, nor that it recognises the potential for helping residents of different cultures feel cared for and at home. Younger Black people may be over-represented in Homes yet their staff teams may have only one or two Black members.

A COCOON IS NOT FOR LIVING IN (NOT FOR LONG ANYWAY)

It is essential that residential Homes do not create some idealised little cocoon of care in which residents are shielded and cut off from the injustices of the wider society. While there are certainly residents (particularly young children) who will need a period of all-enveloping care, such provision must be part of a longer-term plan for growth and independence.

We are most aware of the harsh, impersonal and brutalising aspects of institutionalisation; but there is another apparently benign and protective way in which Homes can operate. Those Homes in which there are no differences of opinion and no arguments, where politics and religion are not spoken of for fear of upsetting people, are the same homes in which issues of race and gender, of low pay and poor housing, of failing social services, of crooked politicians and 'fat cat' industrialists, and of private or public health are seen as irrelevant to the lives of the residents. In these Homes you will probably see no newspapers being read (except in the staff room) and a pretence that it is all a very bad and dangerous world out there. The managers of these Homes will argue that a monthly staff meeting is more than adequate to sort out any minor difficulties, and that residents can have their 'little committee' as often as they wish to because they like to plan the menu and outings. Such homes feel claustrophobic and stultifying.

This sort of institutionalisation suits organisations. Such homes often get excellent inpection reports and residents, having been gently coerced into polite compliance, all report how kind the staff are and how well they are looked after. 'Difficult' residents are avoided and if, by some mistake, they manage to sneak in, they are very quickly eased out again as soon as it's evident that they don't 'fit in'. The same goes for staff.

A TIME OF HOPE

'Living a life' is always complicated. Things rarely work out for any-one in an ideal way. Residents of Homes have had more complicated lives than most people and the decision (however arrived at) to come to live in a Home always marks a time of massive complication for each person involved. Coming into care is usually a time of great loss, but may turn out to be a time of change and hope. The purpose of residential care is to provide services, support and a therapeutic context in which people can live their lives. For some this will be 'living out' their lives; for others it will be preparing to move on, growing up, finding more independence, gathering strength, kicking a damaging habit and leaving something behind. But it will always be complicated. It is useful – even heartening – for staff to remember that helping people with their complicated lives is their job. It is not their job to ignore, deny or remove those complications. The temptation to try to establish a perfect system – a cosy little cocoon, a risk-free and smooth-running institution – is great; but such a system meets staff (and residents') needs to isolate and protect themselves from life's complications, rather than accepting that residents (and staff) bring with them a tangle of difficulties and dilemmas, of hopes and aspirations.

Chapter 9

Staff

The grand old Duke of York . . .

i The most important and expensive resource: the work-force
What do the regulations require? – The costs of staffing and their effect
on the costs of care – Attitudes to staffing – The principles of staffing –
The staffing costs of Norwood House – A radically different way of
managing staff

ii Managing the organisation of staff
Recruiting and selecting staff – Creating a structure to support and guide
the work – Rotas

This chapter is the most directly practical in the book so far. The
examples set out in Part I – with their extensions in Part II and in
the previous chapter – are practical in a sense (because they describe
what actually happened and how managers managed in a wide variety
of situations), but as yet there has been little direct guidance. While
managers need to understand the principles of design and must build
their own systems accordingly, there is practical advice to be given
about matters of recruitment and selection, organisation, communication and supervision. An abundance of useful literature is readily
available (which will be referred to). This chapter will not simply
summarise or repeat what is available, but build on it and, continuing
with our examples, we will see how some of our managers dealt with
staff and staffing.

The most important and expensive resource: the work-force

WHAT DO THE REGULATIONS REQUIRE? (HOW LONG IS A PIECE OF STRING?)

The regulations state that the organisation running residential Homes (that is to say the 'person registered' or the 'responsible authority') must: 'employ by day and, where necessary, by night suitably qualified and competent staff in numbers which are adequate for the well-being of residents' (10 (1) (a) of the *Residential Care Homes Regulations* 1984); and 'ensure that the number of staff of each children's home and their experience and qualifications are adequate to ensure that the welfare of the children accommodated there is safeguarded and promoted at all times.' (Part II, 5 (1) of the *Children's Homes Regulations* 1991). In other words you must 'ensure' that the piece of string is long enough and strong enough to go around the parcel and to secure it. Fortunately there are many authoritative guides and much official and near-statutory 'guidance' issued over a long period (some of them predating the above regulations) which broadly agree how long and strong the string should be for specified parcels. Since 1991, when local authority inspection units were first being set up, inspectors have been specifying the minimum levels of staffing which are acceptable for each sort of Home. They have based these minimum levels on the recommendations of *Home Life* (Avebury 1984), which in turn had drawn on *Staffing Ratios in Residential Establishments* (Lane 1980). Eleven years earlier *The Residential Task in Child Care* (known as the *Castle Priory Report*) (Castle Priory Study Group 1969) was most pioneering and influential in making careful, precise calculations – instead of ill-informed rough guesses – for staffing requirements in children's Homes. Following the publication of *A Positive Choice* (known as the *Wagner Report*) (Wagner 1988) the Wagner Development Group produced *Staffing in Residential Care Homes* (Wagner Development Group 1990), which uses the same methodology as and builds on the earlier Residential Care Association (RCA) recommendations (Lane 1980). The briefest and simplest exposition of staffing figures appears in *Home Life*, and very few inspectors, managers and planners have even heard of – let alone read and understood – the previous publications. Without the knowledge of how and why the *Home Life* figures were arrived at, they are of limited usefulness on their own. This relative ignorance has allowed some organisations running residential care to hoodwink inspectors and care managers into accepting inadequate staffing.

The problem about relying on 'received' staffing figures rather than on figures worked out from first principles is that they are inherently inflexible. Managers really need to understand the principles of staffing, rather than simply implement a formula. No matter how well you have learned a set of figures, knowledge of the numbers alone will be inadequate for the design (or redesign) of an organisation as complex as a residential Home.

THE COSTS OF STAFFING AND THEIR EFFECT ON THE COSTS OF CARE

We have already explored the implications of under-resourcing residential care. The two alternatives of 'engage' or 'disengage' have been spelled out, and nothing pushes a Home more inevitably down the path of disengagement than insufficient and inadequately trained and experienced staff (see Chapter 8, p. 91).

People who have no direct experience of working in residential care – and even some who have but have never had to struggle with designing a rota – find it very difficult to believe the sheer numbers of staff needed to meet the requirements of the regulations – to be 'adequate for the well-being of residents', and to be 'adequate to ensure that the welfare of the children accommodated' is 'safeguarded and promoted at all times'. Managers (and inspectors and planners) need to carry in their heads useful 'rules of thumb' with which they can do very quick calculations of staffing needs. In a Home for older people, for instance, you are going to need about one member of staff (including domestic, catering and management staff) in post to provide for one resident. In a Home for children and teenagers, or for people who have severe disabilities, you are going to need two workers for every resident. You can then do a very quick sum based on what you might be paying the average workers in the Home and include the cost of employing them – say £15,000 a year per person (a little under £300 a week); now you have your starting point for how much each place in your Home will cost (see Chapter 11). This is why there is great resistance to considering the real costs of staffing a Home properly, and why very few Homes are in fact staffed properly. When the cost of staffing alone starts at a level way above the fees which local authorities are willing to pay for the residential care of older people, policy- and decision-makers prefer to remain ignorant and to pretend that the permitted levels of fee are adequate. Generally they are not. Older people in particular are being short-changed by receiving care which often costs a quarter of the fees which are charged for a child or young person, and can sometimes even cost as little as an eighth of the fees of a specialist children's Home. In such 'cheap' Homes, you can be sure that either there are too few staff or they are being paid a pittance, or – most likely – both.

ATTITUDES TO STAFFING

The outsider, typically a local authority social services or voluntary organisation committee member, or a director or senior manager of a private care company, looks at the establishment lists for Homes which are adequately staffed and asks, 'Why so many staff? When I went there on Monday evening there were only two staff on duty. Where were all the others?'

Confronting these critics with the staffing 'requirements' as set out in *Home Life* or in the inspection unit's standards is not likely to change their attitude. But because they may themselves work in an office – quite possibly in the headquarters of some sort of 'human service' organisation – the following step-by-step thought process may help them to understand the basics of staffing residential Homes:

First imagine that your office must be staffed from 8 a.m. to 10 p.m. – twice as many hours as you now have to cover. Therefore you will need twice as many staff. Then imagine that you must staff it throughout the night as well – from 10 p.m. to 8 a.m. the next morning. That entails another shift of staff – a long shift of ten hours. It must surely be obvious now – before we add further requirements – that already you must have three times as many people to provide one person on duty as you needed before you were required to keep your office working all round the clock.

Next, remember that a residential service has to run every day of the year and that you cannot make do with skeleton staffing, because the needs of residents don't reduce at weekends and holiday times; indeed, they may well increase. So add another 112 days to be staffed – getting on for 50 per cent more than the maximum of 253 days which you staff in your office – with three shifts to cover on each of those additional twenty-four hour days. Then add the need for vastly more coordination – 'handovers' between every shift, supervision, team development work, etc. Staff working at night or at weekends will require time to meet with other staff working different shifts, and to work in conjunction with you, or other people like you, who work from nine to five, Monday to Friday.

You will not, of course, forget that these residential workers are entitled to the same length of working week (thirty-five hours?) as you are, and that they, too, will have days off, holidays, periods of sickness, compassionate leave, time for training, days in lieu of bank holidays, etc. If you have thought it through, and have been doing some rough calculations as you go, you may now have realised that it will take about six people in post to ensure that a Home has one person on duty around the clock, 365 days a year. And if you now look at the staffing figures for the Homes for which you are responsible, you will be concerned that they may be seriously understaffed.

A very different attitude is called for from those who plan and manage residential care. In the current fiercely competitive climate, when all the different organisations providing residential care are trying to undercut each other, and the 'commissioners' (purchasers) of the services are haggling for lower fees, staffing – by far the most expensive resource – is constantly being pared down. A higher proportion of agency, 'bank' (see p. 195) and other temporary workers is being employed rather than having adequate establishments of permanent staff. Instead of planning and calculating their staffing on the basis of sound principle and the needs of residents, some private providers are looking to inspection units to tell them what is the minimum they can get away with (Burton 1997). Unfortunately some inspection units (under the improper influence of their local authority colleagues who are 'buying' these cut-price services) then re-interpret and twist the regulations and guidance, and allow Homes to be inadequately staffed. (See Chapter 15).

THE PRINCIPLES OF STAFFING

First – and most obviously – staff are employed and deployed to give care: to meet the assessed needs of residents as specified in each resident's care plan. Therefore we have first to calculate the needs of residents in terms of planned, individually given care, group care, and care which is available when needed but is not exactly predictable. The last category will include reliable responses to individual events and changes such as bereavement, illness and loss of mobility or continence, to minute-by-minute unpredictable needs like wanting a drink or a sandwich, wanting to be helped to the toilet or to read a letter, or attention to sudden emotional upset. So, when planning the work-force, you must try to quantify predictable needs of all residents individually, and then build in a generous and realistic allowance for all the other needs for immediate attention which people will inevitably have.

Residents' needs

Each resident has a unique requirement, but rather than spend a lot of time and effort calculating every resident's exact requirement of staff time it is possible to adapt already researched and established figures. These figures are those used in *Home Life* (Avebury 1984), which themselves were taken from *Staffing Ratios in Residential Establishments* (Lane 1980), which in turn were derived from research carried out by the Social Services Liaison Group Working Party (British Association of Social Workers 1978)! It should be borne in mind that this research was conducted more than twenty years ago, when the population of residential Homes was much less dependent than it is now. Nevertheless, these are the figures which were well researched at the time and which, through *Home Life*, have been used to set staffing standards ever since (Table 9.1):

Table 9.1

	Hours required per resident	
	Per annum	Per week
Mentally ill	416	(8)
Low-dependency 'mentally handicapped' adults	312	(6)
High-dependency 'mentally handicapped' adults	676	(13)
'Physically handicapped' adults	780	(15)
Elderly physically dependent	572	(11)
Elderly mentally infirm	676	(13)

(The wordings of these categories reflect the time when they were written.)

The research was originally conducted when thousands of people who would now be in residential Homes were considered to be too dependent and were therefore in long-stay hospitals, and thousands of other less dependent people, who would now certainly be living in their own homes or sheltered housing, comprised the main population of residential Homes. It is also very important to note that the research considered only the physical care needs of residents. It is reasonable to place most residents (of any age) who have multiple disabilities or a major frailty such as Alzheimer's disease in the highest-dependency category – 780 hours. Clearly fresh research is needed. (It was disappointing that the new standard-setting text, *A Better Home Life* (Avebury 1996), which was so detailed and comprehensive in most areas, failed to update these figures.)

Having added up the care hours required by all the residents, the next step is to divide that total by the number of direct care hours which each full-time staff member can provide. The figure of 1,500 hours per year is set out in *Home Life*. (This in turn is based on the figure arrived at in the RCA (Lane 1980) document.) However, now that a thirty-five- rather than forty-hour week and twenty-five days' annual leave are common conditions of service, the total available direct care hours would be about 1,300 hours per year.

Some progressive inspection units have adapted and updated the *Home Life* figures to take partial account of the greater dependency of residents. For instance, the London Borough of Camden Inspection Unit's Code of Practice (1993) specifies:

Homes for seventeen or more elderly people: a minimum of thirteen day-care hours per resident per week.
Homes for seventeen or more elderly mentally frail people: a minimum of fifteen day-care hours per resident per week.

Every manager of a residential Home is responsible for providing adequate staff. She or he must work out the staffing required – not simply take it on trust – and must then review it regularly in the light of residents' changing needs. The principles are the same in all Homes, although the requirements will vary with the needs of residents, and the size and task of the Home and/or its units.

Let us now apply the adapted *Home Life* figures to one of our homes, Norwood House (Chapter 4). (What follows is an account of the process by which Rachel, the manager, and Lok, her manager, planned the staffing of the resource centre.)

Assume that out of a maximum of 75 residents, 40 are in the lower- and 35 in the higher-dependency categories.

40 (residents) × 13 (hours per week)	520
35 (residents) × 15 (hours per week)	525
Total	1,045
× 52 (weeks per year)	54,340

Divide this total by 1,300 (direct-care hours per care worker, 35-hour week, 25 days annual leave)

Number of day care staff required (to nearest whole-time equivalent)   *42*

or

Divide by 1,500 (direct-care hours per care worker, 40-hour week, 20 days annual leave) Number of day care staff required (to nearest whole-time equivalent)   *36*

When planning and proposing staffing, it is important to calculate on the basis of what 'should be' and what you may have to 'settle for'; so it is important to be aware of the 1,500 figure if the worst comes to the worst.

(Readers will have noticed that the detailed figures so far have been based on the needs of older residents. The figures for younger people are different but the principles are exactly the same.)

Having established the total hours required and divided that by the available staff hours (1,500 or 1,300) and thus calculated the minimum overall number of staff needed, a further, complementary calculation must be done to calculate the number of staff needed to provide the right number of people on duty (often referred to as 'cover'). By making both these calculations, you will have attended to both the sum of individual needs and the whole group/Home needs. The higher of the two results (usually 'cover') should be adopted as the minimum because staffing must meet both requirements.

'Cover'

In a Home or part of a Home (a 'group living unit') where residents need to be lifted (requiring two staff) or where two or more residents may regularly need urgent and immediate attention at the same time, there should be at least two members of staff on duty during the day. Obviously, if the group is small, two may be sufficient but for greater numbers more are needed. Estimating staffing cannot be an exact equation because residents' needs are in part unpredictable. You must add to your careful assessment of predictable needs both the possibility of emergencies such as fire and your educated guess about likely combinations of other unpredictable circumstances. (Such circumstances are well illustrated by the example of Mr Brown in Chapter 8, p. 91.) Therefore when you estimate the staffing for a Home or a unit of a Home, you must be thinking of how many staff you need to 'cover' these eventualities as well as how many you need to attend to specific and predictable tasks. You must also consider the social ambience of the Home. If staff are working non-stop to attend to predictable and unpredictable needs of individual residents, they have no time to sit and talk, to have a sociable cup of coffee with residents, to chat and gossip. Staff create the atmosphere (it's part of their job) and they must have time and opportunity to do this. On the other hand, the presence of too many staff just waiting to 'pounce' on residents' slightest hints that they need assistance is oppressive and institutionalising.

Home Life gives 'rule of thumb' figures of the number of staff you need in post to 'cover' having one person on duty:

> 3.5 full-time workers are needed to provide 1 member of staff on duty during waking hours.
> 2.5 full-time workers are needed to provide 1 member of staff on duty during the night.

Each 'group living unit' and the respite care unit at Norwood House can accommodate up 15 residents, but in practice no unit usually has more than 13. This 'under-occupancy' is due in part to there being two larger rooms on each unit which are big enough for a couple to share; however, it is very rare to get two people who choose to share. Most of these larger rooms are used by residents who like the extra space for a wheelchair, and for those who like to spend a lot of time in their rooms and treat them as a small flatlet. (Since the refurbishment all the rooms have en suite bathrooms.)

To care for an average of 13 less dependent residents each unit will require a minimum of two care staff on duty during the day and one at night. On the units for more dependent residents three staff will be needed during the day and one (with recourse to immediate backup from another) at night.

Therefore the care staff establishment at Norwood House is as follows:

> *Two less dependent units*
> 2 staff on duty in the daytime $\quad$ $3.5 \times 2 = 7.0$
> 1 staff at night $\quad$ $2.5 \times 1 = 2.5$
> A full care team of $\quad$ 9.5
>
> *Two more dependent units*
> 3 staff on duty in the daytime $\quad$ $3.5 \times 3 = 10.5$
> 1 staff at night $\quad$ $2.5 \times 1 = 2.5$
> A full care team of $\quad$ 13

Respite care unit – staffed to the same level as the more dependent units

A full care team of   13

This provides an overall establishment so far of:

$2 \times 9.5 = 19$

$3 \times 13 = 39$

Total $= 58$ day and night care staff

Other staff

Each group living unit will need domestic support throughout the week. This can be provided by having two part-time (0.75 of a full-time post – 26.25 hours) domestic care workers. They will then be able to work 'opposite' each other, i.e. working alternate weekends and mornings and evenings. There will be a domestic care worker available for some part of every day but they won't 'cover' the whole of the waking day. They will both be full members of the care team and very much part of the unit. They will often help with the care of residents because at Norwood House the false demarcations between jobs have been abandoned in favour of working as a whole integrated team (see the example of Ellen on p. 56).

2 part-time domestic care workers for each group living unit

Total   10 domestic care workers

In addition to the group living care staff teams, there are several other teams to be established: catering; laundry, public areas and handyperson; day centre and social, cultural and educational events; and the management team.

The rationale for staffing these teams is more straightforward than for the group living care teams. Of course, with most of them there is a need for a seven-day-a-week service, but not for a twenty-four hour-a-day service. Also, they are smaller teams, which makes their coordination easier. At Norwood House these other teams were as follows:

Catering

2 cooks and 2 kitchen assistants   4

Laundry, public areas and handyperson

3 domestic workers and 1 handyperson   4

Day centre, and social, cultural and educational events
2 day centre/activity workers and 1 community/outreach
worker   3

Management team
4 assistant managers and the resource centre manager   5
                                                          Total   16

THE STAFFING COSTS OF NORWOOD HOUSE

The total staffing of Norwood House (including day-care and community resources and outreach) added up to eighty-four posts, a few of which were part-time. It was important to cost all services, especially the residential places. The average employment costs (including employers' pensions and national insurance contributions) in the late 1990s were £15,000 per annum for a full-time member of staff. This brought the 'unit cost' of staffing per resident to rather more than the cost of one member of staff, even before other running and capital costs were added (see Chapter 11). The equivalent of 7 full-time posts could be attached to the non-residential care side of the centre's work (2 day centre/activity workers; 1 community/ outreach worker, 1 kitchen assistant; 1 domestic worker for the public areas; 1 assistant manager and the equivalent of 1 full-time post apportioned to the hours of the group living unit's domestic care workers). The usual residential occupancy was 65 (13 on each of the five units) and so the staffing of each residential place was costing approximately:

> *74 (full-time posts) x £15,000 (average employment costs)*
> (divided by 65 residents) = £17,000+ p.a.

With an average place at the home costing nearly £330 per week just for staffing, the local authority were spending considerably more for places at Norwood House than in the 'independent sector' (private and voluntary). (Places in the other smaller local authority Homes were even more costly.)

Of course, places in the higher-staffed respite care unit and units for more dependent residents were more expensive than in the two other units – by about £77 per week. In these units, however, Norwood House was providing a specialist service for which the private sector would charge much more. The fact was that the local authority purchasers (community care managers) would only very rarely pay more than £300 for a residential place, no matter how dependent the client was, but they would pay up to £400 if residents were assessed as being in need of a nursing Home.

Lok and Rachel were under great pressure to reduce the staffing in order to achieve more modest 'unit costs' (cost per resident). The costs on the other group living units at Norwood House were considerably less because they had smaller staff teams. The assistant director (Lok's manager) had done some sums and reckoned that if all the residential units were staffed at the minimum level permitted for less dependent residents (which is what the 'competition' was doing for all residents), and if volunteers ran what he considered to be the 'extras' of day care and the other 'fancy bits' of the resource centre, the overall staffing could be cut by about twenty. Also, in his view, the home was perpetually under-occupied because nearly all the double rooms were being used as singles. The occupancy levels could go back up to 100 per cent – or seventy-five residents. The assistant director's sum was as follows:

56 (full-time posts) × *£15,000 (average employment costs)*
(divided by) 75 residents = £11,200+ p.a.

This would bring the average staffing cost per resident down to roughly £215 per week – less than two-thirds of the current average costs. He also had ideas for reducing some of the part-time hours and for recruiting new staff at lower salaries, and his idea for reducing night staffing by using video surveillance would push down costs even further. He reckoned that, with 'realistic' management, he could get the staff costs down below £200 per resident.

The local authority which ran Norwood House had committed itself to a devolving and decentralising management strategy (Chapter 4, p. 30). 'Cost centres' were a key concept in the strategy. Distinguishable units of service, like residential Homes, would have their own budgets and should 'sell' their service to 'purchasers'. While, to begin with, no funds were actually transferred between purchasing and providing sections, the 'cost centre' should manage its finances as if it were an independent unit having to bring in at least as much as it was costing to provide the service. Rachel (the manager) saw great advantages in this process and thought it was particularly suited to running a large 'resource' centre like Norwood House. She felt it gave her the freedom to manage the Home, to be more entrepreneurial, to make local contracts and negotiate innovative funding arrangements, and to take full responsibility for staffing and funding. She also involved staff, relatives and residents in discussions and decisions about the budget. Lok, too, approved of it and had worked steadily with Rachel to implement what they both had eagerly welcomed as a serious and fundamental change of direction for the social services department.

The new 'strategy' was based on the comprehensive review and recommendations made by a large firm of health and social services consultants, who had also recommended the development of resource centres, such as Norwood House, which could give a wider and more flexible service to pensioners and would form part of a network of support services. The local health authority had originally contributed 25 per cent of the conversion costs of the building and had seen its success as integral to its own plans for ensuring (with the social services department) that there was adequate community support and care for older people throughout the area. Its immediate concern was that there would be a range of suitable accommodation and care for older people whom it was discharging from hospital – a concern which local GPs and the health service trusts naturally shared. On the other hand, having 'jointly funded' the conversion of Norwood House, the health authority felt there should be no need of further support, especially as it was now itself ruthlessly cutting huge swathes of the community health care provision which it purchased from health service trusts, and from various private and voluntary organisations. Since the 'joint funding' of the building work at Norwood House, the health authority had had very little contact with the local authority's senior planners and managers, through whom such joint endeavours would usually be created.

Using their own initiative but with the – somewhat shamefaced – agreement of the assistant director, Lok and Rachel had gone to visit the director of community care commissioning at the health authority. They put it to her that Norwood House would no longer be able to take the higher-dependency residents (for whom they had a well-deserved reputation of providing excellent care) if the staffing levels were reduced. They needed some sort of 'top-up' to bridge the gap between the staffing costs of the lower- and higher-dependency residents. The director of commissioning was sympathetic and wished that she could do something but the health authority's current joint funding (with social services) of residents in nursing Homes was stretched to its limit, and was itself under threat. It could not provide top-up funds for places in any residential Homes (even though, she conceded, Norwood House provided a better service to residents who would otherwise be in nursing Homes). It was even contemplating withdrawing the funding it was currently giving to residents in nursing Homes which it used to manage directly but which were now run in 'a complicated arrangement between a community health care trust and a housing association (see Chapter 5, p. 35, and Chapter 12, p. 195). She realised that if those homes then closed through lack of funding – and their places cost £700 a week, of which the health authority paid about £300 – it would need Norwood House even more.

Rachel was not prepared to compromise further on staffing. With Lok, she had designed the staffing at Norwood House to do the job. There were certainly not too many staff, nor were they overpaid. Originally, Rachel and Lok had planned to have more staff, but they had trimmed the numbers on the two units for less dependent people in order to bring down costs. If it hadn't been for the enthusiasm, exceptional teamwork and flexibility of staff, the low levels of staffing on these units would have been inadequate. They were providing a very high quality of care to residents and such care cost a lot of money.

Having never fully accepted or understood the concepts of devolved control and 'cost centres', the assistant director intended to intervene. The only message which he had understood from the consultants' recommendations was that Norwood House would have to 'compete' with the independent providers which – he knew perfectly well – had cut staffing below the minimum requirements. If Norwood House did not 'compete', he would find a way to close the place. Closure was an attractive option because of the huge saving which could be made without cutting any other service. He reckoned that a place at Norwood House would soon be costing £450 a week, and total running costs would be about £1.5 million a year.

Yet the sheer numbers of staff at Norwood House – larger than those in any other service unit in the department, combined with their 'arrogantly independent attitude', made the prospect of trying to close the place daunting. He would love to get shot of them and reckoned that their obstinate response to the video surveillance proposal and their failure to prevent a resident (Mr Brown) from wandering opened up opportunities for attack.

A RADICALLY DIFFERENT WAY OF MANAGING STAFF

What was it about the staff team at Norwood House which made it such a threat and a thorn in the side of the assistant director? What distinguished the group of Homes of which Jeeva was manager (Chapter 5) from all the other Homes which were run by Janet's housing association? What was it about practice at The Drive (Chapter 2) that changed so radically after Sonya left and Bob arrived? What methods did Marcia employ to create a good experience for residents at the Una Marson Project (Chapter 1), even when the weekend's arrangements were so shambolic? And what was the essential ingredient of the recipe which Noreen (Chapter 3) 'just knew' and which Thomas both knew and understood, that enabled The Limes to be such a good Home? In each case it was a special sort of management.

We have dissected and examined some of the component parts of this special sort of management in Chapter 6 (pp. 55–61) where, by analysing the way in which a member of staff (Ellen) engaged with and responded to a resident (Paul), we considered organisational structure. We looked closely at roles, responsibilities and boundaries, and built a structure in which each worker (and each resident) could be clear about his or her own job and its relation to everyone else's, and the team's responsibility for the primary task. Now we will look at how good management enables such a structure to work.

Managing the organisation of staff

RECRUITING AND SELECTING A STAFF TEAM

In the first part of this chapter we followed the complex process of planning the staffing for Norwood House: up to eighty-four staff, split into five care teams and other management and support teams. And in Chapter 3, we saw how Noreen and Reg, after many years of successful informal recruitment of staff, planned a new, formal recruitment and selection process when appointing their new care manager. We have considered the ways in which organisations may use the selection of staff to achieve covert objectives: by, for instance, appointing Bob (Chapter 2) as head of a Home which the senior managers want to close.

Although Noreen and Reg recruited care teams which were an excellent mix of different, talented people, they didn't know quite how they did it, and they were consistently lucky. However, when they recruited Thomas, their new care manager, they used a consultant to help them to work out exactly what they were looking for, and, having been successful in getting the right person for the job, they were then very ready to acknowledge that a well-thought-out, formal recruitment process could be extremely effective.

The long-winded, bureaucratic processes used by the local authorities which ran The Drive and Norwood House, and by the housing association for which Janet and Jeeva worked, were at the opposite extreme from the informal methods generally prevailing at The Limes. Recruitment in these organisations suffers from being a specialist area handled by the 'human resources' section – or, as it used to be known, 'personnel'. The direct responsibility is (wrongly) removed from the manager of the service and is taken by personnel specialists who may know very little about residential care and the sort of staff and teams who are likely to do it well.

The result is often 'block' recruitment of staff, using inflexible methods of selection which are insensitive to the needs of the specific Home and its residents, and which ignore the very different tasks, work cultures and objectives of Homes. A general advertisement is placed for staff of various grades and shortlisted applicants are interviewed for jobs which have a common person specification even though the vacancies are in very different Homes. The procedure is, in fact, just as haphazard as Noreen's old method – but, generally, far less successful.

Following repeated scandals and enquiries into abuse and malpractice, a committee chaired by Norman Warner was commissioned to report on the selection, development and management of staff in children's Homes. The committee reported in 1992 and made excellent, comprehensive recommendations for new good practice. (The report, *Choosing with Care* (Warner 1992), is usually known as the *Warner Report*.) Warner and his committee surveyed the widely different recruitment and selection practices, and distilled the best practice, rejecting the long-winded and obstructively bureaucratic, and adding practical recommendations for innovation. The recommendations of the *Warner Report* are easily adaptable to all kinds of residential work, but very few organisations have got near to implementing them in full. As so often happens with such reports, after the approval, discussion and hurrahs have died down, there is a widespread belief that all the identified faults have been corrected, but the recommendations of the report are allowed to sink steadily into oblivion.

A statement of purpose and objectives; a job description; a person specification

When recruiting staff your intention is to find a particular person whose particular skills, experience and personal attributes make her or him the right person to do a particular job in a particular Home. Even before advertising, you have to be clear about the primary task of each Home, the way in which that Home is run to perform that task, and the contribution that the person appointed will be required to make. When you have clarified these basics (which must be clear not only for recruitment purposes but for running a Home at all), you will then be in a position to specify the details of the person who will be suitable for this job (to draw up a 'person specification').

Advertisements and application packs

Having worked out these essentials, you are then in a position to draft an advertisement which will attract the best available person for the job. It will tell potential applicants what they need to know and enable them to decide both if the job is suitable for them and if they are suitable for the job. It may seem an obvious point, but you should avoid attracting applicants who don't want to do the job and/or are unsuitable for it. The ideal advertisement for a job will be so framed as to elicit replies only from candidates who can be shortlisted. In other words, they should in a way shortlist themselves before sending for an application form. Certainly, the application form and the information you send with it should put candidates in a position to judge whether this is the job for them or they are the people for the job.

The information which you send out in the application pack should of course include the person specification – telling the candidate what you are looking for – and full, honest information about the organisation, the Home and the job. You do not want to waste your own time or the candidate's on applications which are based on misleading information and are later withdrawn, or, much worse, lead to an appointment in which the successful candidate discovers that the job is not at all like the one she or he had envisaged.

You should tell prospective candidates what the timetable of selection is and exactly how you will draw up the shortlist. If you are not necessarily going to shortlist everyone who meets the person specification but, depending on the volume of applicants, shortlist only those who best meet the specification, you should say so at this stage. The more straightforward you are with candidates, and the more open and clear you make the shortlisting process, the better. You are establishing a relationship – and a contract – both with the person whom you will eventually appoint and with an important group of people who are also suitable (though not this time successful) and who may well apply again or have other dealings with your organisation at some time in the future.

Selection

Your shortlist will of course be made by comparing what candidates offer in their written application with what you have said you require in the person specification. Having made your shortlist – selected those people you want to see (who may be the best of many who meet the specification) – you can then test those requirements of your specification which are fairly easily testable. In most jobs – certainly in all management jobs – in residential work, you will need people who can think, write and speak clearly and handle figures. Competence in these areas can be tested.

For some posts you may decide to use personality testing. If chosen carefully, these tests will point to areas of strength and weakness, and to particular traits (such as emotional stability) which can then be followed up in interview.

You will need expert help with testing aptitude and personality. The tests (and your evaluation of them) must be relevant to the job and fair to the candidates. For instance, the tests should not discriminate against people from minority cultures (and many have been criticised for this in the past). They should be geared to people from a wide variety of cultures and backgrounds; indeed, through written tests you may be able to discover candidates' awareness and knowledge of various cultures, which you will then need to follow up in interviews.

Part of selection (and self-selection) should be a visit to the Home and meeting residents. Residents of all ages and of a wide range of abilities can also make a judgement about the suitability of candidates. Just like staff who are involved in selection, they too must have training and support for doing this job, and they should get some sort of formal recognition for taking part in the process. (This might be done by paying them a fee or offering them the choice of a meal out or an outing instead of payment.) Their involvement should be carefully planned and should be given a specified weighting in the whole process of selection. All candidates who have been shortlisted should make the visit and be assessed by residents.

Using references: an important part of the selection process

It is common practice for local authorities to take up references only after the successful candidate has been chosen at interview and then offered the job 'subject to satisfactory references'. By adopting this procedure, selectors deny themselves information which could assist them in making the right choice. References should be taken up when you are compiling the list of candidates to be interviewed at the final stage of the selection process. By studying references before actually interviewing candidates, you and your colleagues on the selection panel will be able to engage them in fruitful discussion of issues arising from their references and thus learn much about their attitude to and suitability for the job you want done. Both before and during the interview you will need to make a judgement of the references – and of the referees too – bearing in mind, for example, that a reference supplied by a previous employer (who no longer has a vested interest in retaining or getting rid of the candidate) can be more illuminating than one supplied by the candidate's current employer. As we saw in Chapter 3 (p. 25), references have an important part to play in the selection process, provided they are assessed with insight and intelligence. What appeared to be a poor reference from Thomas's previous employer was interpreted as quite the opposite by Noreen, and had the effect of recommending him for the job.

Complex jobs which attract a large number of suitable candidates may require two stages of shortlisting. The first stage may be referred to as 'longlisting'; the second stage will lead to a final interview of what should by now be a small number of candidates, all of whom are suitable for the job. The task at the final interview is to use all the evidence which has been collected from the selection process so far, and through questioning of and discussion with the candidates, to make a final selection of the very best of a good bunch. It will be much more revealing to talk with candidates about what they have in fact done and what their ideas are for the job in question, than to ask them hypothetical questions about what they would do 'if'. Interviews should be revealing discussions, not simply question-and-answer sessions in which a good memory and careful preparation are used to achieve 'high marks'.

Equal opportunities

Like the principles and values of good care, equal opportunities policies (EOPs) can easily – and frequently do – become institutionalised to the point that they are no longer liberating and strengthening, but constrict-ing and oppressive. They are too often experienced as procedures in which personnel staff and managers are 'expert' but which the people who are actually managing a service find negative. It is common to hear managers saying, 'Oh, we can't do that because of EOP' rather than 'We can now get the staff we want because of EOP.' An equal opportunity policy, properly understood, internalised and implemented, should give a very strong positive message to all involved – employers, employees, candidates, people who use the service, and the general public. When designing a recruitment and selection process, managers of Homes will not feel constrained by a good equal opportunities policy, but assisted and supported by it. Through it they will get the best person for the job.

We have come across many examples of equality issues in our stories about managers. Residential care is always full of them. The Una Marson Project (Chapter 1), where Marcia worked, was initially aimed at Black women, but as it became established it became a multiracial Home with a mixture of clients and staff (Black and White). (Although, at this early stage, the project was for Black women only, it did in fact have a very wide range of clients and staff from many different cultures and Black ethnic backgrounds. So, to some extent, the project was already multiracial and multicultural.) To begin with, it was able to advertise specifically for Black workers (under Section 5 (2d) of the *Race Relations Act* 1976) and only for women workers (under Section 7 (2) (e) of the *Sex Discrimination Act* 1975). Later, when the culture and ethos of the Home was strongly established and Black clients knew that their needs would be met, the Project opened its doors to White women clients and dropped its policy of having an exclusively Black staff team. As long as there was no danger that the project would become a predominantly White service in which Black clients would begin to feel excluded, there were great advantages in maintaining a fully mixed clientele and work-force. (Because the project was a service for women, many of whom had been in violent and abusive relation-ships with men, the policy of recruiting women workers only was continued.)

The process described at the Una Marson Project – of an established Black service becoming a multiracial service – does not usually happen the other way round. Homes which are White in the majority of their staff and in broad culture tend to stay White. Even when organisations' equal opportunity policies ensure the recruitment of Black staff, the Home can still stay White! There are many Homes for older people in local authorities and in the private and voluntary sectors which may even have a majority of Black staff but the culture of the Home continues to give a message that Black residents are not welcome and will not get suitable care and consideration as an ordinary part of the whole service provided for them. At best, Black residents may be given patronising special attention and at worst they will meet with hostility and indifference. While such a large proportion of Homes remain incapable of meeting the needs of Black residents, there will continue to be a need for Homes aimed particularly at a Black clientele. 'White' Homes can certainly become multiracial and multicultural, but the transformation requires a concerted, long-term commitment from all the staff. It will require White staff to appreciate that they too are different in a team which values people's diversity, all of which can be brought together so that the differences in fact contribute to a whole service (see Chapter 12, pp. 186–95).

Noreen (Chapter 3), a White, working-class Irish Catholic, who had herself had long experience of discrimination, was lucky to have Black colleagues and friends to start up the Home with her. Without consciously pursuing an equal opportunities policy, The Limes was a place where there was genuine equality of opportunity. Staff and residents brought a variety of cultures, races and abilities to the place – from the start. They valued each other's differences. Diversity made the place what it was. When Ann, a person with learning disabilities, got up and chaired the meeting (p. 109), she was taking an opportunity; she was using her abilities; she was relishing her equality as a respected human being living in a community of very different but equal people. It was no accident that Thomas, an African man, got the job as manager. He selected the place and the people as much as they selected him. He selected The Limes for its atmosphere and special – almost tangible – culture. He did not select it for its equal opportunities policy. Like Lok (Chapter 4), Thomas had worked in a local authority which, in straining to promote equal opportunities for all through cumbersome and oppressive procedures, had unwittingly trampled on many an individual's opportunity, while leaving untouched the narrow-minded bigotry of several senior staff (such as Lok's manager).

CREATING A STRUCTURE TO SUPPORT AND GUIDE THE WORK

You have planned your staffing and selected your teams; now they need a structure which will support and guide them. The structure will be a complex but carefully constructed network of interlocking relationships. These relationships are built up from and woven around the primary task. We know that a staffing structure which is modelled on the bureaucratic hierarchy of the larger organisation will not work for residents. In Chapter 6 (pp. 56–61) we saw how a suitable structure had been created in a small team. We will now look at particular aspects of that structure under three broad headings: staff support and development; the organisation of work; communication and coordination.

Compartmentalising these three parts of a complex structure is intended to help us to analyse the complexity. Figure 9.1 is a way of envisaging the relationships between the primary task (giving care) and the organisation of work, the maintenance and development of staff, and the coordination and communication necessary to apply the staff to the job.

The two lower overlapping circles represent the two broad categories of managing staff which are essential to giving good care – even if only

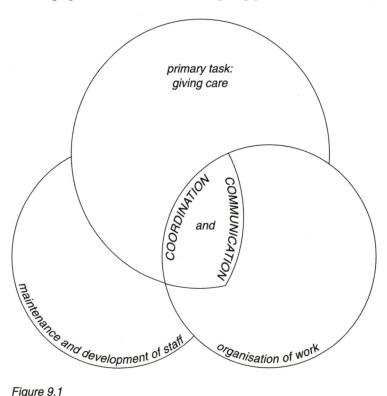

Figure 9.1

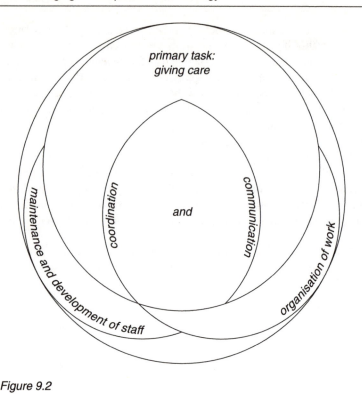

primary task:
giving care

maintenance and development of staff

coordination

and

communication

organisation of work

Figure 9.2

one person is doing it. But as we have seen already from the immense complexities of staffing a Home like Norwood House, coordination and communication are the key to doing the job properly, and this applies to the smallest Homes as well.

When Homes are well managed the processes represented by these circles are integrated. That could be illustrated by the circles being almost on top of one another – within the same circle of good care. Staff support and development and excellent organisation coordinated by a constant flow of purposeful communication produce good care (Figure 9.2).

When the management of Homes is breaking down, these circles shrink until they don't overlap at all. There is no communication and coordination at all and there is precious little care given (Figure 9.3).

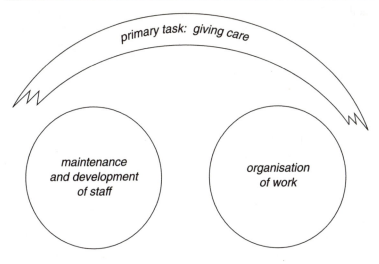

Figure 9.3

Staff support and development

Residential work is emotionally, intellectually and physically demanding. It draws on the whole of a worker. All workers at every level need training to equip them for doing the job, support to maintain their resources for doing the job, and development so that they can advance the work of the Home and their own careers.

Putting training in context

External training for residential workers now consists of a hotchpotch of short courses (many of them geared towards obtaining National Vocational Qualifications (NVQs)) and a few excellent post-qualifying and advanced courses. Most residential workers have no directly relevant qualifications at all and therefore NVQs, which are awarded when candidates demonstrate their 'competence', are a welcome development as an opportunity for staff to gain formal and transferable recognition of their skills and experience. NVQs are a very important development and offer the only currently available hope of establishing a basic, non-professional qualification. However, in spite of the laborious efforts of the Central Council for Education and Training in Social Work (CCETSW) to establish and assure quality in preparation for and assessment of the award of NVQs, the standard varies from good to poor. It is another field for the 'quick buck' privateers, some of whom advertise for trainees in local papers and use a combination of employment and training grants to run schemes which can, and often do, exploit both the trainees and the residents of the Homes in which they are placed. In some schemes, trainees pay a fee to the agency in the hope that they will gain both a job and an NVQ at the end of their 'course'. The 'course' consists of unpaid placements in poor Homes and a few training sessions. The 'training' company may argue that it is preparing trainees to be assessed, but often the preparation is woefully inadequate and the company turns out to have no formal access to or connection with an assessment centre. Of course, this is the worst end of such training but even in some of the formally accredited schemes standards are very low.

In most management jobs in residential care, employers specify that a qualification is required. However, there is no current professional qualification specifically for residential social care, so employers often list all the old professional qualifications (going as far back as the 1950s) and the current social work qualification, the Diploma in Social Work (DipSW). The post-qualifying and advanced courses (particularly in child care) provide experienced and qualified practitioners and managers with important opportunities for further learning. There are very few of these courses and they are expensive. Some Diploma in Social Work courses were temporarily adapted to incorporate residential child care but this has only happened since the *Utting Report* (*Children in the Public Care*, Department of Health 1991) recommended this change. Warner (1992) proposed that there should be a distinct, new diploma for residential child-care workers, but there has been no active response nationally to this more radical proposal, and there has been no corresponding recommendation for training in other areas of residential care.

At least there has been some discussion (and some half-hearted implementation through the 'Residential Child Care Initiative' – the temporary DipSW adaptation) of proposals for qualifying training in the residential care of children and young people. However, diploma-level, professional training in residential work with other client groups is not seen to be important. For work with most other client groups there is no expectation that staff (other than managers) will be professionally qualified, and any qualification – teaching, nursing or social work – is seen as a bonus. Even managers of Homes are rarely qualified through the Certificate of Qualification (CQSW) or Diploma (DipSW) in Social Work, let alone through the – now defunct – specialised residential work training of the Certificate in Residential Social Work or the (later) residential option of the Certificate in Social Service (CSS). The absence of qualifying training and the belief that residential child-care adaptations to DipSW courses are adequate reflect the lack of involvement and commitment at political, academic and senior managerial levels. Residential care is by far the largest, costliest and most staff-intensive of all social-care provision; in addition, it makes the most complex intellectual and emotional demands on staff, yet it has no qualifying training to fit people to become residential care professionals.

Even mediocre residential Homes will be inundated with requests for 'placements' of students on DipSW and many other courses. But if a Home is not yet providing induction for new staff or regular and reliable supervision for existing staff, how will it give a good placement to a student? Although it is the job of student placement officers to ascertain that a placement is suitable, they are so desperate for places that most will not want to hear about the deficiencies of the Home. In addition, a manager – therefore a potential student supervisor – may be seduced by the fees on offer and the prospect of the extra kudos of becoming an accredited practice teacher. This process of accepting a student for placement is similar to that of accepting a new resident when you know that you are failing all the current residents and would fail the additional resident even more. If you already do one, you will very likely do the other.

It is within but in spite of this demoralising limbo of neglect that a training culture must be created in the Home. As in all other areas of residential care, change and progress will come about through the inspiration and efforts of residential workers and managers.

Establishing a training culture in the Home

In the computation of available staff hours (p. 122), five days per year for each member of staff was reserved for training (Lane 1980). Since this figure was proposed in 1980 as an average allowance, it should now therefore be treated as a working minimum which all staff should see as a right. As with supervision (see p. 143) the provision and take-up of training opportunities should be an integral part of the job. Training will include mandatory courses on such basic matters as food handling and safety (for anyone – and that should be everyone – who handles food in a Home), lifting physically disabled residents, and fire precautions. It will include 'in-house' training provided either by members of staff themselves or by outside trainers who visit the Home and work with the staff team. It will include outside training for staff, some of whom may be working towards qualifications such as NVQs or advanced certificates, diplomas or degrees. All training should be relevant to the life and work of the Home. Therefore a training programme showing both individual and team training should be on view for inspection by staff, residents and visitors.

Although to begin with it is likely that the Home's manager will lead the way in establishing this culture, another senior member of staff may be able and willing to accept the challenging role of 'training coordinator', seeing it as an important part of her professional development. This will be someone who has shown a sustained interest in her own training – an enthusiast – and she will probably also become the 'workplace assessor' for NVQs or the 'practice teacher' for DipSW students on placement.

At staff meetings there should be a regular training update and a slot when people who have been doing training report back to their colleagues. If a member of the kitchen staff goes on a Caribbean cookery course, that should be seen as quite as important (as it is) as a senior worker going on a course on advanced supervision.

As the training culture becomes established, all staff get involved. Supervision; planning; engaging and responding; reviewing and evaluating every aspect of work present opportunities for reflective learning through practice. The Home and its work are the core of training activity. You will have to turn down nine out of ten requests for student placements so you will be able to take your pick. It will become widely known that merely to have worked at such a Home will guarantee a substantial level of skill, competence, knowledge and good experience.

Such training 'on the job' should be planned, evaluated and formally recorded, and this can be done through a 'personal development contract', another Warner (1992) recommendation.

The personal development contract

The contract should be the nucleus of staff development, training and appraisal of progress. Just as residents need formal plans for their care (care plans), which assess their current needs, plan how those are going to be met, and review and evaluate progress; and just as each Home should have its development plan, using the same process of assessing, planning, doing and reviewing; so individual staff should be able to make progress in a planned, methodical and formally recorded way.

Induction and supervision

The first period of training, development and supervision will be induction – for everyone moving into a new job, whether they are new to the Home or whether they have changed jobs within the Home. Induction programmes should be based on the individual needs of each member of staff and the job he or she is doing. Clearly there are common areas of induction for everyone, such as all aspects of safety within the building, but different jobs and people will have different emphases. The particular 'package' which is chosen for individual new workers will be determined by their initial assessment with their supervisor.

Further development is built on the foundation of a good induction. In staffing terms, managers will have to remember that initially the effect of each new member of staff will (and should) be to make more work not less. If given proper induction – for at least two weeks – a new care worker is not going to be in a position to add to the available care which the Home provides, and she or he will also take up a considerable amount of the time and energy of other staff.

Supervision starts with induction. During their first week, new workers are likely to need short meetings with their supervisors every day in order to understand and process the mass of information which they will have picked up. The induction period is so important for creating expectations and meeting them reliably. It should be clear to all members of staff that they will receive supervision regularly and reliably. The supervision provided for individual workers will be focused on: their direct work with clients (i.e. giving care); their ability to manage their own work within the organisation; and their own personal support and development (Figure 9.4).

Group supervision and consultation

In addition to individual supervision, it is important for staff to become aware of, reflect on and analyse the processes which are going on in the team, in the resident group, and in the whole community or household of the Home. This is best done in staff group meetings in which consideration of the relationships within the group itself will point to the content and meaning of relationships in the Home. The goal is to engage and respond. Awareness of the dynamics of the group and the interrelatedness of the staff team with the residents and of the residents with the staff enables the team to take responsibility for and to change

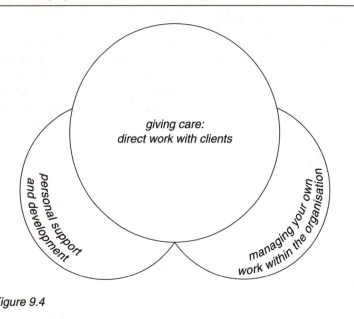

Figure 9.4

ways of relating which would otherwise remain unconscious. If these powerful unconscious forces are not recognised and worked with, staff very quickly become only reactive and defensive: colluding, punishing, ganging up, withdrawing and blaming, to the extent that they eventually become quite unable to engage and respond.

Some Homes employ an outside consultant to help the staff group to do this difficult and vital work. Many Homes which realise the need for such work to be done are not given the resources to use a consultant, yet may manage somehow to do it. There is a danger that a team may get into a rut with a consultant who has been with them for years and, between them, they allow the meetings to become the only time when underlying issues and the unconscious group processes are discussed. Under these conditions, meetings become self-indulgent diversions from the task.

There are warning signs that consultation meetings may be becoming counterproductive. Members of the team appear very clever and perceptive in their observations and criticisms of almost everything that is going on, but they remain uncommitted and inactive about changing anything. It suits them to work in a dysfunctional organisation; but they are part of it. Often, the managers of Homes and the ancillary staff – even if invited – will stay away, and attendance of other staff will be patchy. A consultant worth her salt will not get drawn into but will challenge these collusions against the task.

Most outside managers still remain unconvinced that such staff group work is at all necessary, especially in work with older people and adults with learning disabilities which is often considered to be uncomplicated. However, even if there is no money to employ an independent consultant to facilitate the meetings, the work may still get done if the manager and staff within the Home are keen (see Chapter 12, p. 187 for ways in which Jeeva provided consultation as an outside manager). Establishing regular supervision and the sort of learning culture which has so far been outlined will inevitably lead to all staff having a heightened awareness of unconscious processes within the team. Even if a separate session is not at first established, Homes with an established learning culture will find a way to do the work, or at least some of it, in training sessions, handovers and staff meetings – whenever they meet together.

Staff meetings

The staff meeting should be the fulcrum on which all the other aspects of the team's work is balanced, and, to change the metaphor, it should be the fountainhead – the source – of each week's work. Because of the inbuilt barriers to communication in residential work (shift work, a large work-force, different teams, a constant and copious stream of information to be processed and passed on) it is essential to have regular and frequent meetings.

It is at staff meetings that the ethic and culture of a team are established. The meeting is a microcosm of the work of the whole Home. Meetings demonstrate (or reveal the lack of) discipline and purpose. Until a Home reaches the stage which The Limes had reached (p. 109), of having community meetings at which the big decisions are taken and the important issues are discussed, staff meetings will be the most influential and powerful grouping. And it will only be through full participation in effective staff meetings that staff will gain the experience and discipline of sharing responsibility, and will thus be prepared and able to allow community meetings to take precedence.

If the staff meeting is always chaired by the manager of the Home, or in her absence the next most senior member of staff, it will be limited in its scope. It is unlikely to progress beyond an information, direction and consultation session, and will certainly not enable staff to begin to share decisions and management with residents. Chairing the meeting is a skill which has to be learned both from observation of others and from the practice of chairing the meeting oneself. Ann (at The Limes, p. 109) learned by watching, listening and taking part in a democratic culture (even though the meetings had not been formal), and by having a go herself at chairing the first more formal community meeting. She was then teaching other people, including staff.

Staff meetings need an agenda and minutes. Simple procedures which formalise but do not constrict are important. (Practical arrangements have to be worked out – among them timing, seating, comfort, agreements about how the chair is elected and how decisions are taken.) It is useful to allocate time in each meeting to the same elements as we identified for structuring work and for supervision (see Figures 9.1 and 9.4). The meeting can then function as the forum for the application of staff resources to the primary task. To function effectively it must itself stay to task:

giving care – concentrate on residents' needs
organisation – concentrate on managing the work together
support and development – concentrate on staff and team training, on reflective and analytical discussion about the state of the Home, and on learning together as a group.

If this structure for the meeting is allowed to slip – most typically if the meetings fail, week after week, to discuss the needs of the residents' themselves – this is a sure sign that defences against the anxiety engendered by the direct work – giving care – are becoming institutionalised. At the same time it would be likely that staff meetings would become introspective ('navel gazing') or repeatedly focused on the shortcomings of the outside management and organisation, or constantly complaining about residents and their relatives, or superficial and jokey, avoiding serious discussion or disagreement. A three-point structure helps the meeting – and therefore the Home – to stay to task.

In any Home it is difficult to deploy staff so that everyone (except those who need to be with residents, or who are on leave or sick) can be at the staff meeting. In a very large social care centre like Norwood House (see p. 91) it is even more difficult. But until managers at all levels understand the significance and central role of the staff meeting in residential care, and accept that full attendance is vital, Homes will continue to fail in their complex and demanding task.

This is yet another area of residential care bedevilled by the ignorance, prejudice and lack of good experience of so many managers and planners.

Lok's manager, the assistant director, was shocked to learn (p. 95) that sixty staff were attending the full staff meeting at Norwood House on the day that Mr Brown went missing. (Of the total establishment of eighty-four, two posts were vacant; ten staff had worked the night before or were due to work that night, five were on leave, two were away sick, and five others were looking after residents on the units.) He was furious that so few members of the large Norwood House staff were with the residents for the hour-and-a-half duration of the meeting; and, in any case, he regarded a staff meeting such as this as being a gross waste of money. He reckoned that each of these fortnightly meetings was costing approximately £750; and nothing in his experience enabled him to understand why they were necessary. None of the other Homes had all their staff on duty for a staff meeting. In those Homes, if staff wanted to come to a meeting when they were off duty, they were not discouraged, and they took the time 'back' whenever they could. He wasn't able to imagine how such a meeting could be effective, for, he reasoned, most of the much smaller meetings which he had to go to – and many of which he chaired – were a complete waste of time.

Effective staff meetings set the tone for all other meetings in a Home. There should be 'handover' meetings every time one group of staff hand over the work to another group: three times a day – from night staff to early day staff, from early day staff to late day staff, and from late day staff to night staff. Again, even though the time is much shorter – fifteen or twenty minutes may be enough for a 'handover' – there should be a regular structure at the centre of which are the residents. Care workers will be handing on their work to others, providing them with information about residents – what they've done and how they are, minor alterations to care plans, changes in medication or diet – and with ideas and observations about residents' moods, anxieties and particular needs. This passing-on of information must be done quickly but carefully; it will therefore require a methodical approach. There will also be some discussion but that, too, needs discipline. Issues will inevitably arise which should be discussed elsewhere. If there is no other appropriate forum (like effective regular staff meetings) then the efficacy of handover meetings is subverted because their immediate and practical purpose is displaced by discussion of and decision-making about major issues.

ROTAS

At the heart of all management there lies this problem: how best to apply the available resources to the task? Designing a rota – often regarded as a mundane operation – is, in fact, a searching test of a manager's capacity to meet that challenge. No Home works as well as it should without a good rota; but in Homes of all kinds rotas are generally clumsy, crude and inadequate. Some follow an unremitting pattern of 'earlies, lates, nights and days off' which could have been derived from hospital practice in the early part of the twentieth century and passed down from one regimented generation of workers to the next. Some follow no discernible pattern at all except that favoured individual staff members are given their own special rotas and everyone else is fitted around them. Some are a chronic combination of the two just described. Occasionally an outside manager will look at the rota in a Home, find it wanting, and, barging through the boundary between his job and the Home manager's, he will come up with a 'new' rota, which he then tries to impose upon a reluctant work-force. 'Of course,' they say, 'he doesn't understand.' They're probably right, he doesn't! But nor do they, and nor does their manager, who should have produced a suitable rota in the first place. As with all other aspects of managing residential care, if you don't understand the principles, you will ultimately fail in the task.

Understanding the principles of rotas

A good rota is a sophisticated, custom-built instrument, not the crude, off-the-shelf contrivance found in most Homes. It is through the rota that the varying needs of residents can be attended to, with higher levels of staffing on some days and at some times of day than others. The rota provides the mix of staff on duty – the right combination of people at the right times. It may be likened to the electronic 'box of tricks' in a modern car – which 'manages' the engine's fuel injection, ignition and exhaust. The rota establishes the underlying cadence, the pulse and the rhythm of the Home. It is both metronome and drums.

In a properly staffed Home, there will be sufficient workers at all levels to perform the primary task – provided they are effectively deployed. While designing a suitable rota, the manager will apply the principles which were used to design the staffing establishment – meeting the residents' needs and providing 'cover'. Add to these fundamental principles all the other facets of staffing which we have already considered:

- 'waking' or 'sleeping in' night staffing
- staff meetings, supervision, handovers
- induction, training, staff development
- reviews, care planning, 'key working'
- annual leave, sickness

and further aspects of staffing which we have not considered in any detail:

- good working conditions and sufficient time off for staff
- equity (but not necessarily exact equality) between all staff
- ensuring that every member of a team works with every other member, thereby avoiding the growth of 'teams within teams'
- 'balancing' the composition of staff on each shift so that there are always suitable people to attend to some residents' special needs – e.g. always having at least one woman on duty in a mixed sex Home.

Like the staffing establishment, the rota has to be designed to provide for most circumstances – the predictable and the unpredictable. The staff team must be self-sufficient and capable of responding flexibly to abnormal circumstances; and yet, because they are working with people whose demands are often unpredictable, staff need steadiness and reliability built into their working patterns. Most residential workers will want to know well in advance whether they are going to spend Christmas Day, Eid, Diwali or New Year with their families or whether they will celebrate their important festivals at work with residents. Therefore the rota has to be reliable and long-term; but, in making it like this, you will build in the potential for flexibility, because people are much more ready to be adaptable from a firm base. Of course, residents also need to know that the rota is reliable – that when a member of staff says she will be with them tomorrow or next week, she will be.

The design and planning of a rota is a difficult and time-consuming task. It must be done by the manager (or a delegated member of the team) of the Home, and not by edict from outside. Any rota will need small alterations each month to accommodate staff changes and absences (a vacancy, annual leave, study days), and all rotas need 'tweaking and tuning' in the light of experience or a gradual change in residents' needs and in methods of work. The person in charge of the rota must check every shift of every day to ensure that the staffing is adequate in numbers and competence; and every worker, when checking her or his own shifts, must also think ahead to ensure that staffing is viable. Although the rota should always be one person's special management responsibility, it must also be a shared responsibility. Because rotas are necessarily complex and, therefore, easy to sabotage, it is essential to consult team members, discuss their work patterns, and be sure that they have a thorough understanding of their rota and are wholeheartedly committed to it.

Chapter 10

The building: the therapeutic environment

I'll huff and I'll puff till I blow your house down . . .

The primary task – What do residents want from a building? – Homely or institutional? – Significant rooms – The office – Keys

THE PRIMARY TASK

When exploring any aspect of managing residential care, we must always begin with the primary task. The sorts of question prompted by the primary task are: What is this building for? Which needs will be met by this room or that piece of furniture? What are we trying to say to people by the way we arrange the front door and entrance? Consider the kitchen, for example. Obviously, it must be designed in a way that enables the cook (or anyone else who is cooking) to produce good meals – nutritious, tasty, well-presented and safe. It must contain the right equipment for the job and it must meet food safety and hygiene standards. If it produces the meals and meets these standards, the kitchen may be judged to be just fine. But will residents' needs – in the fullest sense of that term – be met? Will the kitchen be a central part of the therapeutic ecology of the Home, or will the food merely amount to high-quality 'in-house catering'? Many managers will be relieved to know that the food is good and will expect no more; and it may also satisfy many residents most of the time. But what else might we expect the kitchen and food to provide for residents? What about their emotional, cultural and identity needs? Will these be met merely by the operation of an efficient kitchen producing excellent food? It is not difficult to appreciate that food has a symbolic value as well as a nutritional value. Feeding, for a new-born baby, is more than nutrition.

Eating, for the child, adolescent and grown-up of any age, is more than a bodily necessity. When Marcia (Chapter 1) managed the barbecue, she had more in mind than nutrition. The meal which she helped residents to prepare was an event of deep social, emotional, psychological and therapeutic significance, and it was at the centre of one resident's belief that this was 'one of the best days she'd ever had'.

Of course, when designing a Home either as a new building or as a conversion of an existing building, the architect will use the requirements, advice and guidance of many different publications and experts. The building must have a minimum number of bathrooms and lavatories depending on how many residents will live there; it must have a minimum area of floor space to each resident for sleeping, sitting and dining areas; it must have fire exits and precautions. There are many features of design for a residential Home which a family dwelling does not have to have. There will be equipment and procedures which are compulsory in a Home but unheard of in an ordinary home – sophisticated fire alarm systems and testing procedures; valves to control the water temperature to protect residents from scalding themselves; cleaning equipment and substances which must be used, stored and accounted for in ways which far exceed the requirements of an ordinary household.

When the architect and planner discuss these issues with the senior manager who is responsible for commissioning the new or converted building, all the 'hard' requirements – those which, although time-consuming and expensive, are relatively straightforward to comply with – are planned into the design. However, as the design takes shape, the obligation to meet health, safety, hygiene and building regulations may be pursued to the detriment of the Home's primary task. The difficult challenge for the manager is to use the regulations to support the primary task rather than allowing them to be the sole or prime considerations in the design.

Senior managers who use their imagination and experience will consider how the new building will be used. They will be aware that the kitchen has the potential to be the 'heart' of most Homes, that food is more than physical nourishment, and that bathrooms must not only contain the right equipment but that they must also be warm, comfortable and attractive. Having done their homework and read the books, e.g. *A Better Home Life* (Avebury 1996), most managers will in fact incorporate such prerequisites in the architect's brief, but many Homes will still emerge as buildings which started with the statutory requirements and were only then adapted to residents' needs. Ideally, the design of every Home starts with residents' needs. The framework of regulation is then used to ensure that the building can meet those needs safely.

WHAT DO RESIDENTS WANT FROM A BUILDING?

Let us stay with kitchens and consider what the needs of children and young people at The Drive (Chapter 2) were.

In the years when Sonya (Bob's predecessor) was manager of The Drive, Ellen (the domestic care worker) was a full part of the care team and took the lead in the cleaning of the Home and the cooking (see p. 56). All staff did their share of 'domestic care' (and also expected residents to help). Although Ellen cooked and cleaned more than most other members of staff, her management of the domestic care in the Home was equally important. She was the person who was 'most responsible' for making sure that the Home was clean and the food was good. She also organised other people and took the lead in integrating the domestic work of the Home with the overall therapeutic task.

Ellen was particularly keen on making the kitchen work well. This was the source of food which symbolised and 'carried' the other good things which could be got from the kitchen. When children came home from school – indeed when they came into the Home at any time – they went straight to the kitchen to get something to eat and drink. Of course, they were often hungry and thirsty. (Such appetite in growing children and teenagers is a healthy sign, both physiologically and emotionally.) But they were also hungry for relationships, contact, affection, appreciation and reassurance. It was not difficult for Ellen, Sonya and the other staff to understand that this repeated homecoming ritual (which most of the children created for themselves and to which staff responded) had strong connections with infant behaviour. These children wanted to be (symbolically) held and fed. Particularly after a difficult day at school, or playing football, or hanging around with friends and getting involved in trouble (or avoiding doing so), or after a stressful visit to their family, they needed a reliable, comforting base to return to and the Home had to find symbolic ways in which they could ask for and get what they needed.

If Ellen was in the kitchen preparing the evening meal, she would usually have made some buns, a cake or some fresh bread. She would also make herself a large pot of tea (more than enough) and would check that milk and juice were ready for anyone who wanted them. She encouraged other staff to do something similar and to have their own 'trademark' – some speciality to offer the returning residents. She made sure that there was a small stock of part-baked bread in the freezer, as a stand-by for those less skilled staff who could neither bake nor come up with another idea. The 'specialities' of particular members of staff were really only a small part of what was on offer to children on their return to the Home, but as Ellen explained to her colleagues, it should be something fresh, something which has been made specially for them, and, ideally, something they can smell as soon as they open the front door and come in.

The kitchen was arranged so that there was space for people to sit round the table and for cooking to go on at the same time. Children liked to see what was being prepared for the evening meal, which one or two of them would usually help with later.

The 'experience' of this kitchen was a central part of the help and support which residents got at The Drive. The kitchen – for preparing and providing good food, eating and being well fed, swapping the day's news, being welcomed home – was at the core of the therapeutic social ecology of the Home.

It is perhaps easier to understand the deep psychological significance of food and the kitchen for children than for adults. Children are chronologically closer to infancy when, as we all know, feeding has deep significance. Yet 'eating disorders' in adults, particularly in famous women, are headline news, and most people understand that such 'disorders' are psychological. Similarly, the other most sensitive, intimate, instinctive and potentially threatening (and potentially deeply satisfying) areas of living – excreting, keeping clean and caring for the body, sleeping and sex – are, like eating, of huge psychological significance. These areas are all concerned with what we take into ourselves and what we put out – concerned, that is, with our bodies as entities, as outward images, 'expressers', containers and protectors of our very selves. Therefore the rooms, equipment and furnishings which are intended to meet these psychological and physical needs must be designed and used with great thoughtfulness and care.

Analysing the role of the building and all that is in it in this way may sound far-fetched and over-complicated, yet Ellen's approach to making such highly sophisticated home-coming provision was no more than she had done for her own children in her own home twenty years earlier. But in residential care what may appear to come naturally and needs no painstaking thinking-through in your own home requires analysis, planning, coordination and management, and there is less room for failure in a residential Home. Having carefully set up the sort of after-school welcome home we saw in our example, failing to provide it might be disastrous for a child in the Home, whereas children of the same age to whom such a welcome (or similar provision at other times) was an ordinary, established part of family life would have already internalised the psychological strength to shrug off the occasional failure, and happily make their own buns – or do without!

HOMELY OR INSTITUTIONAL?

When designing the building and its contents, some planners and managers are aware of their psychological significance and their potential for therapeutic care. Consequently they strive to achieve a 'homely' rather than an 'institutional' result. So, while the design of the main kitchen at Norwood House, in which meals for over a hundred people were produced, had of necessity to be institutional, the design for the kitchens on the group living units was much more homely. Small Homes such as the Una Marson Project and The Drive had homely kitchens; and, although it was a much larger Home than either of these, The Limes also had a very homely kitchen. But, as we have seen in the example of Ellen's use of the kitchen at The Drive, the homeliness of buildings and particular rooms is produced by a combination of both the physical attributes and how they are used. There are many examples of Homes into which homely features (e.g. group living units) have been planned but where the use that is made of them is highly institutional and institutionalising. And there are many other examples of institutional buildings which lack homely features but which are transformed by the non-institutional approach of the staff.

Architects are famous for getting it wrong. The walkways and 'villages in the sky' of the 1960s' and 1970s' municipal housing developments were good ideas which generally failed. These were carefully thought-out attempts to 'build in community'. Having commissioned their idealistic estates, local authorities made the mistake of thinking that 'community' was created by the buildings themselves, rather than by the way people used the buildings and lived in them. Similarly, there have been many good ideas from planners and managers about how residential Homes should work, which they attempted to build into buildings but which were never made to work. The philosophy and practice will utilise, shape and adapt the physical provision – whatever it is.

While Sonya and Ellen (Chapter 2) would probably say that the most important room at The Drive was the kitchen, Bob would almost certainly say it was the office: same building, but a different philosophy and practice – and a different primary task. In use, the building and its contents will express the dominant philosophy and practice. The physical provision is part of the therapeutic (or anti-therapeutic) language of the place; just as there is 'body language', so there is 'building language'. A skilled and experienced observer will be able to discern where the Home is on a scale ranging from 'homely' to 'institutional'.

Much will be revealed simply by observing what rooms are called; what notices (if any) there are on doors; which doors are locked, which are left open, and which are knocked on; who uses which rooms; how information is displayed; what pictures, books and ornaments there are around. Open or closed, doors will betray much information, starting with the front door. Notices and pictures will also be a mine of information to the practised observer and, perhaps less consciously, to the visitor or new resident.

Table 10.1 compares homely and institutional names for rooms, and for other parts of the building and garden. Those marked in the 'Institutional' column with two asterisks (**) are 'out of bounds' to residents and are locked by staff when not in use; those marked with one asterisk (*) are used by residents only when accompanied by staff and also locked when not in use.

Of course a Home must have a kitchen! but, as we have already seen, it can be homely or institutional depending on how it is designed and used. The presence of an office does not necessarily mean that a Home is institutional – most Homes need an office – but how the office is used will set the tone. The names alone will not tell you whether the Home is homely or institutional. It will be the cumulative evidence of their names and the uses to which they are put which will indicate how homely the place is. 'Managing' a Home to be 'homely' may sound both tautological and contradictory, but the contrast between Bob's and Sonya's approaches will demonstrate first that a Home can be far from homely, and second that managing does not have to imply institutionalisation.

Homes unwittingly adopt and maintain both the descriptions and the uses of rooms which were established at the planning stage. When an architect writes 'matron's office' and 'food store' on a plan, these names

Table 10.1

Homely	Neutral	Institutional
	Kitchen	
Larder		Food store**
Dining room		Dining area
		Servery
		Snack area
Living room		Lounge
Sitting room		TV lounge
		Smoking area
		Games room
		Recreation/rumpus room
Hall		Foyer/reception
		General office*
		Manager's office**
		Matron's office**
Study		Quiet room
		Chill-out room
		Therapy room
		Medical room/surgery*
		Hairdressing room
Backyard	Garden	Play area
		Staff/visitors' parking
Loo	Toilet/lavatory	Ladies/women
		Gentlemen/men
		Staff toilet**
		Visitors' toilet**
	Bathroom	
Cupboard		Store**
Airing cupboard		Drying room
		Laundry
		Sluice room
	Stairs	Lift
		Fire escape
Back door		Emergency exit
		Boiler room**
	Bedroom	Sleeping-in room**
		Staff room**
		Staff changing room**

(and the attitude which produced them) can stick. Using building regulations and guidance, planners may insist on reserving one lavatory for staff, another for visitors, and others for residents (and even they are separated into men's and women's). But for a manager and staff to accept such segregation and its implication of inferiority is to collude with a very institutional attitude, which will seriously undermine all other attempts to create a homely atmosphere.

Homes are very different: different sizes, different client groups, and different purposes. These differences will influence how homely or institutional – overall – they are. In a very large Home like Norwood House, there will be public and sizeable communal areas which must be managed in a way which meets the needs of a large number of users. The large-scale central catering for five separate group living units and a luncheon club must be highly organised if meals are to be produced on time, economically and to a high standard. Neither residents nor staff can be allowed to wander in and out of the kitchen while the cooks are busy. Consequently the homely side of cooking will have to be accommodated and encouraged on the group living units. That is why they were built: to counteract the disadvantages of the size of the Home; to create homely living in a large institution. So Rachel, the manager of Norwood House, constantly supports staff in all their efforts to make the place homely: she takes down the notices, attached to cupboard ('store') doors during the conversion, which proclaim 'This door must be kept locked at all times'; and, as we have seen (p. 95), she explodes in fury when the assistant director proposes installing video surveillance equipment. Even good Homes are a compromise between the ideal of a completely homely atmosphere created to achieve the primary task (which always includes the fundamental idea of providing a 'home', see p. 55), and the inevitable demands of organisation and regulation (meetings, rotas, hygiene, safety, budgeting, etc.), which themselves are intended to support and manage the primary task.

SIGNIFICANT ROOMS

The kitchen has significance because of food and feeding. Lavatories and bathrooms are important because in them people excrete, keep themselves clean (or are helped with keeping clean), look after their bodies and preen or groom themselves. Most people would choose to make these private and solitary activities, but some – particularly older, frail and/or physically disabled residents – will need help.

So, how should we design for, build in and create the right layout, equipment and atmosphere for such intimate and personal places?

Of course, people have very different tastes and needs, but planners and managers can start with their own standards. They can ask themselves what they expect when they stay in a hotel. Do they prefer to have or insist on having an 'en suite' bathroom and lavatory, or are they quite happy to use a bathroom down a corridor, sharing it with other guests (strangers)? They can then make further progress in their planning by imagining themselves to be quite severely disabled – to be slow – to find most bathrooms and lavatories difficult to use – to need help. In such circumstances most managers would surely opt for up-to-date equipment which they could operate themselves when they needed to be lifted, washed and dried. Or would they be happy to have to ask two members of staff to help them – to lift them, to transfer them from chair to wheel-chair, from wheelchair to toilet, then back to wheelchair and to chair, in the meantime removing their lower clothing, wiping their bottoms, washing them and replacing their clothing? Advanced equipment is expensive, of course, but it is not nearly as costly as staff time and back injuries; and it is cheap when compared with the price that residents pay for their loss of dignity and control.

Similarly managers could reflect on their own habits and circum-stances at home. How many toilets and bathrooms do they have? Do they enjoy having a bath? How do they pamper themselves? What makes using the lavatory enjoyable for them? A nice warm room? Something to read? A good view? A cigarette? Soft toilet paper? Security and a bit of peace and quiet? A satisfying result? Perhaps planners and managers would even go so far as to acknowledge that as young people (and even now in their maturity) the bathroom was and is the place for lengthily and minutely scrutinising one's face in the mirror, for exploring and examining every part of the body, for cossetting and indulging, and for gentle masturbation. This is ordinary, natural behaviour which for most people will add to their appreciation of themselves and their bodies. People living in residential Homes may have had experiences and histories which undermine their confidence and pleasure in themselves, and which result in dislike – even disgust – of themselves, their bodies, their sexuality and of other bodily functions. It would not be too great a leap of the imagination for managers to realise that – like them – residents also need clean, comfortable, warm, private, well-appointed bathrooms and lavatories so that they too can indulge in the same intimate and necessary pleasures.

Residential care managers who are knowledgeable and experienced will be able to think more deeply than simply comparing their own needs with residents' needs. They will understand the full therapeutic implications for vulnerable and frail people at any age of carefully designed bathrooms and lavatories.

Bedrooms are the only areas of the Home which residents can (or should be able to) call exclusively their own. Yet many residents are sharing rooms, do not have a key to their room doors, and have staff walking in and out without their permission. While managers should of course take steps to put a stop to such flagrant denials of residents' rights, they will not be very effective until they have examined their own part in such bad practice. The widespread continuation of sharing rooms when residents have not made a clear positive choice to do so brings shame on the organisations – and their managers – which allow it to happen, on the community care managers who place and pay for residents in shared rooms, and on inspectors who turn a blind eye to this outrageous denial of basic rights. There *are* certainly unusual circumstances when two residents wish to share a room, and then their wishes should be granted. But most rooms are not shared by choice; they are shared because residents have been given no realistic alternative. Unless two people are a 'couple', relatives or close friends and want to be together night and day, no shared room can be the private living space to which we all aspire – in or out of residential care.

The bedroom or bedsitting room is the resident's domain. Like a bathroom, a bedroom is an intimate room in which the resident needs comfort and privacy – and, above all, security from the 'perils and dangers of the night' by which, to some degree, we are all threatened. Sleep is a state of unconsciousness. In sleep one is prey to uncontrollable dreams, even to talking or walking without being aware or having any control, and one is very vulnerable. Going to sleep – letting go of consciousness – can be frightening, and yet being unable to sleep and lying awake in the dark can also be very frightening and stressful. Waking up and facing the day is daunting for many people. (And for some residents being in bed or in a bedroom will have terrible associations – amongst them, memories of violence and sexual assault.) Yet, as experience proves, the resident's bedroom can become a haven: a vital component of the therapeutic environment.

Colours, fabrics, pictures and furniture (including, of course, the bed) should express the very personal tastes and preferences of the resident. While it may not usually be possible to decorate and refurnish whenever there is a new occupant, if the resident is expected to have the room for a significant time, very considerable changes should be made to suit her or him. In long-stay situations, residents will often wish to bring their own furniture with them or to buy some special items to suit the room and how they are going to use it. People get even greater pleasure from their own things in a situation where they share so much with other people and where so much is already provided. Having your own TV, your own chair and bed, and your own bedside light and table are very significant symbols of ownership, control and independence. Some older people get great satisfaction from lying in bed, watching television and controlling it with their own remote control. Residents should feel that they have the same absolute control over their doors – over who can come in and when. The contents and uses of the bedroom, like those of the kitchen, are not merely practical contrivances to meet physical needs. They are symbols, indicative of care – of seeking to meet a person's emotional and psychological needs.

Although the furnishing and decoration of a bedroom for children and very short-term residents may be difficult to change to any great extent, significant adaptations can be made which are again of both symbolic and practical value. A child (or adult) may feel safer with the bed in a different position. A resident may not like a picture or may find a large wardrobe frightening. Staff must find out how he or she wants the room and do their very best to change it in the way the resident would like.

THE OFFICE

Offices in Homes are very revealing. We saw in Chapter 2 how Bob's attachment to his computer and office represented his real interests, and how he had deserted the original primary task of The Drive in favour of an administrative task.

As with other rooms, it is not only the physical position, furnishing and equipping of the office which determine the extent of its institutionalising influence but, of course, how it is used and who uses it. Offices are often staff hideaways or even little fortresses. They are places in which staff get away from residents and then build defences against them. A lot of what is done in the office, behind a closed door, could be much better done at a table in the dining room or, in a children's Home at bedtime, sitting at the top of the stairs.

When Janet (Chapter 5) made her extended visits to some of the Homes for which Jeeva was the outside manager, she noticed that offices were used very differently from the way they were used in other Homes. When Jeeva himself visited, he rarely went to the office first, and even when talking with staff or doing any sort of paperwork, he would find a quiet corner in one of the larger communal rooms or, during good weather, in the garden. Of course, if there was confidential work to be done, he asked if there was a private place to talk in, but usually the office was neither private nor quiet so it was unsuitable for the purpose.

Janet herself, when first making these visits, half-expected and half-wanted to sit in the office, for people to come and see her there, and to be brought some tea or coffee. That's what happened in most of the other Homes, where everyone was 'in their place': the office was for managers, professional visitors, senior staff, for other staff strictly on business, and occasionally for relatives and residents if they were being 'seen' in the office. All the administrative, financial and management work was done in the office. If the manager came out of the office, she was seen to be coming on to the 'floor' (the shop floor), but that was not her real place of work. In the Homes which Jeeva managed, people were in and out of the office all the time. The office in these Homes was where only some of that sort of work (office work) got done. It was a central point of communication for both inside and outside matters. It was where the safe and the locked filing cabinets containing confidential information were kept, and it was where the administrative worker was based, but it was not the most important room in the building, nor did association with it confer higher status on anyone.

It was not surprising that Janet felt exposed and uncomfortable at first; she wasn't used to having such direct and continuous contact with residents, care staff and the whole busy life of a Home. Yet as she observed Jeeva at work – on the occasions when their visits to the Home coincided – and saw that the managers of the Homes hardly used the offices, she began to understand what it was about these Homes which was so different. The difference was not, of course, merely in the use of the offices but it was represented by the way they were used. Jeeva and the managers in the Homes spent most of their time with people in the areas where they worked and lived. If Jeeva was in a Home at a mealtime or at coffee-time, he sat down with residents and staff and took part. Without appearing to do very much, he was in constant contact and in a position to monitor all the really important things which were going on in the Homes – and so were the managers of the Homes. Through his consistent example, Jeeva was fostering a very different sort of management. Janet saw that he was working on many levels at the same time, and moving easily between them as if it was the most natural thing to do. Of course it was; but when Janet first tried to do it, she found it exhausting.

She realised that the use of rooms in other Homes – most significantly the offices – in exclusive and hierarchical ways was a means of splitting the work up into separate bits and assigning a higher or lower status to each. This made the work easier but much less effective. It created unhealthy divisions between managers and staff, between groups of staff, between staff and residents, which the rooms then symbolised and reinforced. And it created strong barriers and defences against the primary task, substituting what should have been support functions for the real job of the place – the care of residents.

Janet learned that there was indeed an alternative way of managing the building only by observing it at first hand and experiencing it. Jeeva had tried, without much success, to explain to her what this different method of management was. He had told her how for managers often the start of change could be raising an awareness of how offices in residential Homes are used and misused. It wasn't until Janet had taken the risk of exposing herself to the experience that she gained the elusive awareness necessary for her real understanding.

KEYS

In residential work, keys are generally accorded much the same significance as offices. They are seen as potent (and portable) badges of power, control and exclusion. In institutionalised Homes – where keys are brandished by staff as symbols of 'authority' – management thinking may be summarised as follows:

> No one is to be trusted. Give residents and staff an inch and they will take a mile. Give the night staff the key to the larder and there will be nothing left in the morning. Leave the larder open and the residents will swarm in and clear the shelves. So, assemble a large bunch of keys to nearly every door in the place and that will give you – the person in charge – a form of control. Everyone will have to come to you whether they want disposable rubber gloves, soap powder, a loaf of bread or a pad of paper to write on. This way you will know what is going on in the place and will be able to manage resources all the better. On the other hand, there is something a bit unhealthy about residents who wish to lock their doors and keep their own keys in their pockets or handbags.
>
> Residents don't need keys – ever. Most staff may be given the key to some areas and not to others – temporarily. Managers keep the keys to all locked areas of the Home – always.

This approach to locking doors and using keys is officious, insulting and untrusting; it breeds distrust. It is also often laughably inefficient. Keys are lost; doors are open when they should be locked; keys are left around; the bunch of keys is stolen and a new set is cut (at considerable expense) or locks are changed (at even greater expense); staff take more supplies than they need and hide them somewhere so their work isn't interrupted by the time-consuming and humiliating key routine; keys are mistakenly taken home; locks are forced or doors broken open either because the key cannot be found or because residents (usually younger people) are impelled to smash their way through locked doors which should never be locked (larders). Staff of both sexes (but more often men) walk around fiddling with and flaunting the keys, or wear them, gaoler-like, on special contraptions to attach them to their belts – and this in what should be a 'home'?

Of course, some keys are necessary, but the fewer the better. First you must start with the principle that residents need to be able to secure their rooms, and take control of that security with their own key. Some residents may decide not to use their locks. And for those who may not be able to keep and use a key, staff must make some provision which ensures that the security and privacy of their room remains in their control, whether they choose to exercise it or not. Next, there must be security for residents' private information (files of all kinds) and for money or valuables which they ask to be kept securely by staff. Then, money and valuables which 'belong' to the Home and are for communal use must be properly safeguarded. Medicines, dangerous substances and some potentially dangerous areas of the home (e.g. the boiler room) must be locked up. And finally, expensive equipment and large stocks of provisions must be secured against outsiders. And the effective use of all these internal locks relies on proper attention to the security of the building itself. Security – protection from intruders – is essential wherever you live, but achieving it should not require a proliferation of bars and grills, lights and alarms, and closed-circuit television.

Because a formidable number of keys will be needed in even the most homely of Homes, managers should give serious thought to their use and to their security. Keys which are not in constant use, nor needed for immediate emergency access to locked areas, should be kept in a key cupboard. The cupboard itself must be as secure as the lock of any key it contains – so it would be foolish to keep the safe key in the key cupboard! And it must be efficiently and tidily maintained. A simple method should be devised to keep track of any key which is taken from the cupboard; for instance, each member of staff should have a 'borrowing tag' to hang in the place of an absent key, making it is easy to tell at a glance who has it.

Keys can become the hallmark of a poor Home in which an obsession with inappropriate security results in the proliferation of keys – lost keys – duplicate keys – defunct keys – unlabelled keys. Anyone who has spent just a little time in residential Homes will recognise the signs when locks and keys get out of control: padlocks on cupboard doors; staff carrying large bunches of keys, half of which they cannot identify; broken locks replaced by more padlocks; broken padlocks!; notices giving orders about locking which are ignored; more notices!; open key cupboards; keys being given to residents and staff so that they can open doors which shouldn't have been locked in the first place.

While the details and practicalities of keys are very important, managers must think about what keys represent and about the principles of locking doors. Keys and the way they are handled are a representation of the philosophy of the Home. As with all other physical aspects of a Home, managers must work on several levels of meaning and practicality. The bunch of keys at the belt of a worker conveys a message to the resident; it probably has an unconscious meaning for the worker and this meaning may be expressed in the way he handles the bunch of keys (the keys have a language); the keys mean that doors are locked and the worker holds the power to lock and unlock. (Are they the right doors? Is he the right person?) The keys and their use are a microcosm of the whole Home, which, with thought and imagination, can illuminate many of its complex workings and relationships. As with the kitchen, or the bathrooms, or the office, even keys may be both an area of real concern and an avenue of significant potential change.

Chapter 11

Money, budgets and finance

I had a little nut tree; nothing would it bear
but a silver nutmeg and a golden pear . . .

Market forces – Residents' money – Petty cash – Budgeting within the Home – 'Outside' management and administration and the Home's budget

The purpose of this chapter is to recommend an approach to 'money matters' which will enable managers to integrate the various financial aspects of running a Home with the whole management task – which is, of course, to further residents' wellbeing. We shall consider the unsatisfactory results of current policy and practice whereby control over a Home's finances is withheld from its manager and control over their personal finances is withheld from residents. We shall argue that unless managers are empowered to take responsibility for managing the available financial resources, they cannot do their work properly; and that unless residents are empowered to take responsibility for managing their own money, they cannot live a full life. We shall advocate a radical rethinking of prevailing systems in which central organisations jealously protect their financial dictatorship and regard Home managers as incapable of making any 'big' decisions about their budgets; and in which Home managers, in turn, defend their superior position and regard residents as incapable of handling their own money. Manifestly inefficient, these 'orthodox' financial arrangements call for the reforms summarised in the following propositions, and discussed in detail later:

1 Good budget management is not achieved simply by the avoidance of overspending.

2 Profit-making organisations are not necessarily more financially efficient than non-profit-making organisations.
3 Managers should be in control of the budget of the Homes they manage.
4 Residents (or their chosen advocates or representatives) should be in control of their own money.
5 The power to take financial decisions should be devolved to those who are directly and personally affected by them.
6 Whenever possible, financial decisions should be taken by Home managers and residents jointly.

'MARKET FORCES'

It's now common for managers to be selected more for their professed financial acumen than for their demonstrable grasp of the principles and practice of providing a good service. Often, the assessment of managers' suitability to 'manage a budget' is based on their familiarity with the current financial jargon and the size of the previous budget for which they were responsible. How they in fact spent that budget and whether the users and purchasers of the service judged it to be good value for money are not usually investigated. Frequently, 'managing a budget' is taken to mean simply following already established ways of spending it, and not overspending it. 'Success' and 'failure' in budget management is simplistically estimated in much the same way as Mr Micawber pronounced happiness (success) to lie in underspending his annual income by sixpence, and misery (failure) in overspending by sixpence. In most large social care organisations, whether they are run for profit or not, money is king, yet there is a poverty of imagination and creativity in handling it. Money is wasted – often because of long-established procedures and even because of overcomplicated safeguards against the misuse of money.

Even when undertaken by rigidly following procedure, managing the budget has more kudos attached to it than managing care has. Much-vaunted systems of quality assurance are often geared to measuring 'input, throughput and output', rather than with outcome – how helpful the service was to the user. In most organisations, the more senior the managers, the more likely they are to be primarily concerned with budgets than with the quality of the service which is funded by the budgets. A similar development is taking place in health and education services. In schools, headteachers are being recruited for financial and administrative management, rather than as educational leaders and excellent teachers who also need to be competent in those financial and administrative areas which are parts of their overall job. The quality of education is measured by the crassly simplistic device of exam league tables, not by much more subtle and significant measures of children's actual experience at school. Similarly, the management of residential Homes is rated on achieving a low 'unit cost' and on their level of 'competitiveness in the market-place'.

In earlier chapters, when discussing the motivations of different organisations and their managers we have recognised that some are driven simply by the aim of making money. Others – particularly local authorities – operated for so long in ignorance of what a service was costing and without making realistic comparisons with the independent providers that, when they were forced to 'compete', they had no background of financial analysis or discipline with which to understand and reform their management. Many had allowed residential services to slide into massive – but decreasingly productive – staffing costs. Instead of radically rethinking how services could be provided and paid for, most local authority managers took the easy way out. Using the excuse that union agreements prevented their Homes from being run economically, they handed them over to the 'independent' sector, from which they then bought back cheaper services which were sometimes no better – and frequently worse – than those they had previously run.

It should not be an insurmountable problem to create high-quality residential care services in local authorities which are in fact better and no more expensive than Homes of similarly high quality in the private sector (which have to make a profit). Quite simply, given the equivalent standards to attain, places in local authority Homes (where the profit margin is absent) should cost less than in the private sector. It is depressing to compare the general performance of each sector. Despite their potential financial advantage, public sector Homes rarely provide a good service economically; and in private sector Homes (where the profit motive must prevail) the quality of service is rarely the prime consideration. (It must be acknowledged that there are exceptions to this general picture. In both public and private sectors there are Homes which are run well – economically, efficiently and effectively – in other words, providing excellent care.)

The principal difference between the public and private sectors lies in their respective attitudes to and management of staffing costs.

Local authorities

The lowish wages for basic-grade workers are enhanced by a complex patchwork of extra payments for different jobs and times of work. Generous special leave and sick pay are exploited by workers who have no stake in the financial viability of the Home. Absences are frequent and lead to overwork and overtime for the remaining staff, and/or the additional expense of taking on temporary or agency staff. The 'central management' costs (outside management, administration and personnel), and supply and maintenance costs are often extremely high. The combination of these circumstances with the unwillingness, timidity and impotence of managers to take responsibility for changing them, rather than just giving up, makes for an expensive and ineffective service.

Private care companies

Very low wages (well below local authority rates) are paid to mostly part-time staff who can increase their earnings only by doing extra hours at the same low wages. Casual staff are frequently taken on and just as frequently laid off, and staffing overheads are avoided by steering clear of trades union membership, employment rights and equal opportunities. Companies rarely contribute to pensions, and any special leave is unpaid. Adequate time is not provided for handovers, meetings, supervision and training (although all the brochures will tell you it is). The work-force is constantly changing. Homes operate on a 'minimum cover' basis and are in frequent negotiation with inspection units to reduce staffing. The companies employ very few management staff.

There appears to be an unconscious collusion between the public and private sectors which results in the run-down, closure and transfer of Homes from expensive and poor-quality local authority services to less expensive – but still poor-quality – profit-making services. Although for some local authorities this is a carefully managed implementation of political policy (and therefore a quite conscious process), in others it is an abject failure of management and leadership, and a betrayal of principle and trust. Social care organisations in all sectors (public, voluntary and private) have swallowed the lie that it is the market, the 'law' of supply and demand, which is the deciding factor – almost the guiding principle – in providing residential care or not.

The rule-of-thumb calculations set out in Chapter 9 (where we discussed the logistics and costs of staffing residential care) will tell us that if a private sector Home is adequately staffed, its fees cannot be less than the average cost of employing one full-time member of staff, plus about another third of that to cover all the other ingredients of care. This means that in a private sector Home which employs sufficient numbers of staff and charges fees of £250 per week, care workers are being paid less than £4 per hour. Bearing in mind that such Homes must also meet interest charges on a high proportion of their capital assets, buy expensive equipment, pay for regular maintenance, put money aside for re-investment and improvements and still make a profit, it is obvious that they cannot afford to pay staff properly. They simply do not have sufficient money coming in to meet their fixed costs and overheads and to give staff a decent wage. In fact it is difficult to understand how they even survive; and when you observe that many do in fact survive – and even appear to prosper – on such low fees, you can only conclude that residents and staff are the losers. Why do local authorities use such Homes when they must know that staff are inadequately paid, trained and supported? And why do inspection units not insist that Homes comply with the regulations, guidance and requirements which relate to staff (see Chapter 15)? The answers to these questions are to be found in decision-makers' attitudes to residents and staff of Homes: attitudes which are most plainly evident in their approach to the financing of residential care.

RESIDENTS' MONEY

To understand what the underlying attitudes to money and finance in the Home and in its managing organisation are, it is most illuminating to look at the way residents' money is handled. We will compare two approaches in the Homes which Janet managed (Chapter 5).

Hetherington Housing (the housing association for which Janet was director of care services) managed twenty-four care Homes and four nursing Homes. Like the convoluted contracts for the management of the Homes, the funding of residents' places was also complicated. There were over 300 residents of all ages (over 18) and with a wide variety of needs. Most residents were funded by local authorities' community care money and some, in nursing Homes, were also jointly funded by the health authority. A few residents had lived in the homes before April 1993, when Income Support (residential allowance) was paid by the Department of Social Security (DSS). They continued to have that money paid directly to the housing association. Residents who came to live in the Homes after April

1993 had only their benefits and pensions paid to the association, and the bulk of their fees came from the local authority (and, for some, from the health authority as well) in the form of community care money. An element of the benefits from the DSS was an allowance for the personal use of individuals, but this too was paid directly to the association. The housing association, the provider of accommodation and services, thus controlled all the money of those for whom it was caring – even their personal allowance. It then paid back the 'personal allowance' to those residents who wanted it, but for most residents it kept the allowance until they or their carers actually said they wanted it.

Nearly everyone in the housing association, from the administrator in the finance department to Janet (in unguarded moments), referred to residents' personal allowance as 'pocket money'. So, too, did officers of the DSS, workers in the Home, relatives and even residents themselves. Outside residential care only children have pocket money; inside residential care – even when run by relatively enlightened organisations – 25-year-olds, 50-year-olds, and 90-year-olds have 'pocket money'. It is kept and saved for them, and handed out – sometimes to them but more often to their care workers or relatives – so that they can buy or be bought all the things which are not provided by the Home (and therefore not included in their fees). Those who are lucky enough or insistent enough to get their money will have less than £2 a day to spend on themselves: to buy drinks, sweets, clothes, presents, cigarettes, tickets to the theatre or cinema, perfume, shampoo, biscuits, stationery, papers, books, shoes, stamps, videos, CDs, cosmetics, hairdos . . . to have a bet, to pay for telephone calls, to save for a new television, to have a meal out. The majority of residents who do not get their full personal allowance each week may be given a pound or two but the rest of their money will be 'saved' for them. Many residents are ignorant of the fact that they have any money at all, and when they are given a little bit of their own money or some more major item – new clothes or a television – is bought for them out of their own savings, they believe that they are being given a 'present'. Indeed, at Christmas, Homes generally ensure that every resident has a good reserve of savings so that they can be bought a 'present'. It has been common practice in some Homes to pool residents' savings – of those who were not aware they had any savings – to buy important communal items. Curtains, televisions and carpets are bought from this fund when the Home's budget does not stretch to such purchases.

When Jeeva had started to work for the association as one of the care services managers two years previously, he had been shocked to learn how residents' money was handled. He remembered the struggle he'd had to persuade his former employer (a local authority) to let go of a similar system in the Home of which he had been the manager. He had expected a housing association to be much more enlightened and to adhere to the widely accepted guideline that the providers of services must not get involved with residents' finances. (While this was widely accepted in theory, it was also widely flouted because long-standing bad practice and underlying institutional attitudes impelled Homes to take control.) Inspectors had sometimes intervened in the private sector where, it was thought, the practice could so easily lead to fraud, but they underestimated the institutionalising and oppressive effects in the public and voluntary sectors. It took Jeeva some months to persuade Janet what poor practice this was. Backed by the finance section of the association, she argued that there would be chaos if most residents either took back control of their money themselves or got a family member, friend or advocate to handle it on their behalf. Jeeva pointed out that there were established official ways for people to act on the behalf of residents by becoming 'appointees', by taking 'power of attorney', or for residents' affairs to be administered by the Court of Protection. Having put his arguments reasonably but firmly, Jeeva continued to encounter strong resistance from all levels of management and administration within the association, and from staff in the Homes. Community care managers (social services staff who 'placed' residents in Homes) at first refused to make proper arrangements for them to have an appointee – someone to administer their money with them – in the same way as they would if the resident were going into a private Home. It was extra work for hard-pressed care managers, and since the local authorities and all housing associations had always administered residents' money, they didn't see why they should have all the bother of finding someone else to do it.

Jeeva decided that he would have to ignore this resistance and, guided by clear principles, he ensured that all new residents to the Homes he managed either made arrangements for themselves or had arrangements made for them so that the association was no longer involved in the administration of their money. Sometimes he had to tell care managers that residents could not be accepted until their financial arrangements had been properly made. After a year most residents had bank or building society accounts of their own into which their benefits and pensions were paid, and out of which a standing order was paid to the association. If they wanted cash themselves they drew it from their accounts by whatever means was most convenient. The organisational pressure persisted, but Jeeva pretended that he didn't know what all the fuss was about, because residents were now managing their money in the same way that all the people he had been obliged to argue with managed theirs. (Of course, he knew very well that the resistance he met was rooted in these people's attitudes to residents, whom they regarded as incapable of exercising self-determination.)

More quickly than her colleagues, Janet conceded that Jeeva was right. Although in some ways it was more trouble to make individual financial arrangements with residents, Janet could see that the new system had huge practical advantages as well as being correct in principle. People's money, the saving and spending of it, and the pleasure – and the worry – of managing it became normal parts of people's lives again. Having money in your purse or wallet was a real pleasure. Knowing that you were 'paying your way' with your standing order, even though only a little was left over, gave some respect and power. If you buy something rather than appear to have been given it, you are in a position to demand value for your money, and you're in a better position to complain. Getting a second cup of tea seems like generosity for which gratitude is an appropriate response if you're not paying for it; but, if you are paying for it, you may justifiably complain if you don't get it.

This new attitude to money, both from residents and staff, in all the Homes which Jeeva managed changed lives and relationships, and was just part of the many other changes which took place. There was also a fundamental alteration in the way the relationships between the Homes and the housing association were conducted. They got on to a much more equal footing because Jeeva and, increasingly, Janet were able to foster the sort of mutual respect in which superiority or resentment on either side was absent.

PETTY CASH

The administration and use of petty cash can have a similarly profound influence on life in a Home. The conventional approach is a bit like the 'pocket money' attitude to personal allowances. When Homes are run by a larger organisation, all money is seen to be the responsibility of central managers and administrators. In spite of much talk about devolving budgets, managers of Homes find themselves reporting to junior administrative staff in the central office on piffling matters such as why was fruit bought in the market rather than ordered from the contracted greengrocer? Or why was a packet of pens bought at Smith's from petty cash when the procedure is for stationery to be ordered from central stores? Many managers eventually conform to expectations, and end up asking exactly the same sort of silly questions of their staff. Staff then give up too and conform to expectations by never buying those nice-looking mangoes from the market when they are cheap, and failing to complete full daily notes on residents because the Home (the organisation) has not provided pens to write those notes with. (The stationery order from central office hasn't arrived!)

Used properly, petty cash is part of the therapeutic tool-kit of the Home. A Home needs a good supply of ready cash, in just the same way as most residents will wish to have enough money in their pockets or purses for all immediate, everyday needs. Just how much ready cash is required very much depends on the size and lifestyle of the Home, but we might be concerned about a place where there are twenty residents and there is only £25 to spend on day-to-day necessities and extras. Such a small amount of petty cash implies that nearly all supplies of every sort are ordered, and delivered to the Home on account (which is then paid by the central administration). Apart from the facts that choice is likely to be restricted, that quality is likely to be low, and that bulk ordering is often very wasteful, the opportunity is lost for residents and staff to get properly involved in an ordinary and very important part of life.

Of course, petty cash has to be exactly accounted for. In the same way as a member of staff, when asked by a resident to buy something, must demonstrate to the resident (and, when necessary, to a manager or relative) that she has paid for the item and returned the correct change because she is handling someone else's money, so staff must account for their spending from petty cash. Expenditure must be recorded exactly and supported by proof of purchase or spending (usually receipts). An 'imprest' petty cash account is based on a very simple system. The sum of money – the imprest – of, say, £100 is advanced from the organisation as a float for petty cash spending. Any money taken from the petty cash must be replaced by a 'voucher' for exactly the same sum. The cash and the vouchers should always add up to the imprest amount. As the cash reduces to the point where there may be insufficient to meet everyday spending – in this case to £50 or so – the petty cash claim is made to the organisation by submitting all the vouchers and the account (which sets out the details of each purchase and specifies what budget it is to be set against, e.g. provisions, stationery, etc.). In return the organisation will replenish the petty cash float (the imprest) to the previous level by paying out the exact cash value of all the vouchers. (In a more advanced system, the cash will be obtained directly from the Home's bank account.) Once all staff using petty cash have understood the simple principle on which it is based, they are more likely to use it properly. However, there are many common and persistent misconceptions. One is that petty cash should be a weekly payment of the float; in other words, the staff believe that petty cash is a form of income for the Home – the weekly cash sum to be spent – and if you don't spend it all, you are losing the opportunity. In fact the imprest is simply a means of spending money which is already allocated to various budgets – for instance, food and stationery – and drawn from those budgets each time petty cash is spent. A Home may also have a cheque book with which other larger and more regular bills can be paid (or cash obtained). Whether you pay the milk bill with petty cash or with a cheque, the money will still come from the provisions budget. And even if the dairy's invoice is sent to the central finance office, the amount of the cheque paid by the organisation will be deducted from the provisions budget. If a member of staff or a resident goes out and buys some extra milk from a nearby shop, pays with cash from their pocket, and then exchanges the receipt for the milk for money from the petty cash, it will *still* be taken from the provisions allowance.

Too often regarded as a comparatively trivial and tiresome aspect of residential care, petty cash can become one of the therapeutic and rehabilitative tools of the Home. Residents (and staff) need to handle money; to budget and to understand how budgets work; to appreciate that all money without exception comes from somewhere; and that, when living in a communal household, there are communal implications and responsibilities attached to spending of any sort.

BUDGETING WITHIN THE HOME

To use money well within the Home it must become an ordinary part of everyday life. When the big decisions about money are made by the central organisation (outside the Home) all the empowering potential for the community is lost, and the relationships embodied in outside control over the budget are oppressive. In addition they have a very practical and immediate consequence. When staff and residents have no stake in the good management of the Home's finances, waste is inevitable: they have no reason not to overspend.

With different client groups different levels of involvement and control will be appropriate. Young children will be helped to control their own money, and perhaps introduced to the bigger issues of the Home's budget by participating in the weekly spending on food, or by being encouraged to budget for outings or holidays. If children take part in the shopping (some of which will be done by using petty cash), they will be helped to understand how much things cost, to compare prices, to decide whether some luxuries or special foods can be afforded this week, and, if so, how they might save a bit on other food to remain within the limits.

The annual budget for food should of course be split up into weeks and months. Residents and staff will need to think about the budget, discuss it with each other in meetings, and, whenever possible, make joint decisions. How much should be saved for the Christmas period? Are we making sufficient allowance for higher expenditure in the winter than in the summer, when food prices – especially of fresh fruit and vegetables – rise? Similarly, the heating and lighting budget will be discussed and expenditure monitored in staff/resident meetings. For instance, in June, when the first electricity and gas bills of the new financial year appear to be well within average quarterly spending, it is easy to forget that they will rise sharply in the winter. This is an obvious bit of common-sense budgeting, but some residents may not be used to planning so far ahead and staff will help them to allow for the fact that winter's bills are going to be much higher and to recognise that economy with heating and lighting is just as important in the summer. This is very useful experience and information for those children and adults who will be leaving the Home to lead a more independent life. They will be in a better position to do their own shopping and pay their own bills than if they had not been living in residential care and had not become interested and involved in budgeting. For those people who are likely to go on living in the Home for a long time, being aware of and making decisions on the communal budget is an important part of sharing responsibility and having real influence on real issues.

Residents (and their relatives) as well as staff should be fully aware of the budget for staffing. They are in the best position to know how many staff are needed and when; and, if properly involved, they will have important comments to make about whether there are too many staff at some times and too few at others. Although the staffing budget for most homes will be measured in hundreds of thousands of pounds, this is all the more reason for discussing its management with residents and staff. If they are fully informed and involved, they are well able to discuss the quality of the service, to judge whether value for money is being provided, and to identify areas in which savings can be made in order to increase staffing where and when it is most needed.

A manager should be judged not merely by her or his success in staying within the budget, but by how that is done. When the budget is wholly controlled by the manager it is a comparatively simple matter to avoid overspending; but financial 'efficiency' so achieved in fact costs a great deal. A major opportunity of enabling the residential community to participate fully in community life has been frittered away. It is when the manager and those who live and work in the Home succeed in managing their budget together to provide good service without overspending that the manager is truly managing well. What dictatorial budget control costs by wasting human potential (for learning, developing, acquiring self-respect and respect for others) cannot be quantified in money terms, but it could be seen as the equivalent of a massive overspend.

The budget – and particular parts of the budget – should be regularly discussed at staff, residents' and community meetings. We saw an example of this at The Limes, where residents and staff meeting to discuss the special meal on Thursday evenings (p. 108) considered not only 'Shall we go ahead?' but 'Can we afford it?' and 'How can we afford it?' And at The Drive where – before Bob arrived – Ellen was fully operational as a domestic *care* worker, in the true sense of that term, she was the member of staff most responsible for the furnishing budget, but that did not mean that she was in total control of it. It meant that she was the person who would 'manage' it – plan it, spend it and account for it *with* the residents and other staff.

One simple way of keeping people informed about spending and of involving them, is to draw up a 'bar chart' of the budget and its separate components. Each bar represents the total spending for the year, which can be shaded in to show spending to date. Dividing the bars into twelve (monthly) blocks, makes it easy to see the progress of expenditure; and provided that the chart is regularly updated, overspend and underspend are plainly evident.

'OUTSIDE' MANAGEMENT AND ADMINISTRATION AND THE HOME'S BUDGET

We have seen that managing the budget plays a crucial part in the internal management of a Home. When a Home is part of a larger organisation (and even when the owner of the Home is not the manager and the financial interests of the Home are thereby 'externalised') there is an inevitable tension between 'outside' and 'inside' over money and who controls it. The fashion for 'devolving' budgets and creating 'cost centres' is currently very popular, but often means little more than an administrative reorganisation of accounting, rather than a real shift in power and responsibility. The conventional thinking on budgets is that they are 'naturally' held and managed outside the Home and all that is required from the manager of the Home is to stick within them. To do so is to be a 'successful' manager. But we have demonstrated that the budget is of much more significance than is assumed in this conventional view. Therefore, rather than starting with the assumption that all budgeting starts by being the preserve of central management (the assumption which leads to residents' money being centrally controlled), we should start from the position that it is 'natural' for residents to manage their own money, and for the community of people who live and work in a Home to manage the Home's money (budget) together. We then see that to do any different would not in fact be 'natural', and that there would have to be very good reasons for budgets not to be managed within the Home.

There are many 'not so good' reasons why a true decentralisation is hard to bring about. Administrators in head offices who have traditionally handled all the financial aspects of residents' and the Home's business have usually believed that they are doing a good job in the interests of residents. They like to provide residents with money. They enjoy budgeting for the Home. They, too, get satisfaction in being involved in an important aspect of giving care, and, not unnaturally, they enjoy the power and responsibility it gives them. Taking it away feels like rejection – a lack of appreciation for all their years of taking care of this side of the business. Taking it away may also be taking away their jobs.

Outside managers, too, have huge problems with letting go of the purse strings. On account of the kudos attached to budgets – and the size of budgets – in the status hierarchy of managers, it is unacceptable to most managers to let the strings slip or to pass them on. They find it hard to believe that the person below them in the organisation could possibly be trusted with her or his bit of the budget. (Those who have children may also find it difficult to allow them to take responsibility for their own money as they grow up; and we may guess that they might have had the same trouble with their own parents.) They then experience budgets and finance as the ultimate management test – a minefield which only they can enter. Those who find it hardest to let go are those who have been unable to integrate money as a part of ordinary life – work life, home life, personal life – and may be unfortunate enough to experience it as an overwhelming desire or threat. Of course, few managers will be quite so chronically obsessed, but, if they are honest with themselves, most managers will find that their reluctance to let go when challenged to do so springs, at least in part, from their personal experiences.

The situation itself challenges them. The situation requires that residents and staff experience the ordinary business of 'making ends meet' and learn how to do it. Outside managers and administrators can be very helpful in this process. The handing over of a budget should not be a petulant 'dumping' of responsibility with an implied wish for failure. It should be gradual. Having understood herself or himself in relation to this letting go and handing over, the outside manager will then be in a position to engage and respond at a level which is not punitive and controlling but offers support and aids development. The fostering of responsibility in residents and staff and their success in taking control of the budget will be a resounding success for the outside manager as well. As always, with clarity and self-awareness, and with the primary task in mind, it is not so difficult to put the principles into practice.

Chapter 12

Putting it all together and making it work: the therapeutic ecology in action

Humpty Dumpty sat on the wall . . .

An integrated response to needs – Residents' needs cannot be neatly separated – Chopped-up care – Therapeutic work: bringing the parts together – The survival of a therapeutic ecology in a poor environment

A home exists for its residents; and it should be so managed as to afford them the opportunity of 'living a life' where resources – staff, buildings and equipment, money – are available to meet their individually assessed needs. We have discussed the deployment of each of those resources in Chapters 9, 10 and 11 but, in practice, it is neither possible nor desirable to separate any one from the others. As we have seen throughout the book (starting with the stories of management told in Part I), the issues facing managers at all levels are inevitably related to all three of those broad categories of resource; and this chapter proposes ways in which they can be integrated and managed to create the 'complex living and learning, adapting and changing organism' called for at the beginning of this part of the book (Chapter 8, p. 90).

AN INTEGRATED RESPONSE TO NEEDS

There should be no place, no event, no time when all the interlinked resources of the Home are not in some way engaged to carry out the primary task – to respond to residents' needs. We have identified ways in which management fails when resources are not integrated. Bob isolated himself in his office (Chapter 2) with his computer and his defensive obsession with administration. In Chapter 4 we saw how out-siders, particularly the assistant director, were trying to force single 'answers' on to complex problems – closed circuit television to stop 'wandering' – as if life and work in the Home were a series of unconnected events which could be singled out and 'dealt with' by managerial edict. Janet (Chapter 5), in common with most of the housing association staff, lacked residential work experience and knowledge. Until she began to gather direct experience and to learn from Jeeva, Janet was perplexed by the apparent fixedness of residential care, by the way in which some Homes seemed to be immune to attempts to change them from outside; but she learned to look at a Home as a whole rather than as a collection of individually competent or incompetent staff, and well-managed or mismanaged events. Yet to understand the whole a manager has to focus on the details and then trace their connections with each other, gradually building a picture of the entire life and work of a Home. As William Blake said, 'He who would do good to another must do it in Minute Particulars'; and this is how good residential work is done – first in the 'minute particulars' and then by assembling those details of engaging and responding into a coherent whole. The manager must practise what is popularly known in management literature as 'helicoptering' – feet on the ground, in amongst the details one minute: high up, taking in the whole lie of the land the next.

The need for integrating – bringing together and using together – the resources of a Home is clearest and most urgent in work with children and young people. As with other client groups, but more obviously, children need a whole experience of care, not separated bits and pieces. Our example (p. 56) of Ellen's twenty minutes' engagement with Paul and of her integral role in the staff team (Figure 6.2, p. 59) demonstrates what such a 'whole' experience might be like.

The good experience which Paul was able to take in – to internalise – was provided in 'minute particulars': in small, barely noticeable exchanges, in symbolic interaction, in the warm, reliable presence of Ellen, in her movements and tone of voice. But the minutiae of such work are the fibres of the fine threads which are woven into the whole fabric of care. The pattern and structure had been thought about by the staff team and had been designed so that Ellen was at the centre of the special care which the whole team considered could best be given to meet Paul's particular needs at that time. Other staff were of course involved although, together, they had decided that it would be Ellen who would do the direct work. They were involved even by agreeing to keep out of the way, while Ellen worked on their behalf as an integral part of the team with status and with control over the Home's resources. Had Paul been able to split the good care provision – warm, but not intrusive affection; control; authority; and gentle understanding – which Ellen was able to offer him in a (grand)motherly way, from all the 'bad' things of his current emotional environment, that would have confirmed his hostile view of a hostile world. Without conscious intention, Paul had been setting himself up for confrontations with staff and other residents and inviting avoidances and persecution. By splitting staff (in his mind) into good and bad (mostly bad), by neglecting and damaging himself (tobacco, drink and drugs), by spoiling his own environment (his room) and by rejecting the nourishment of the Home (food and meals) only to 'steal' it later and wolf it down secretly in his room, Paul was taking into himself the same hurtful slights and rejections which he was showing to others. Ellen had connections with and authority in all these areas of grievance, but unlike her colleagues, she had not felt personally attacked and rejected by him.

Paul's situation and behaviour would have been approached very differently if he had come to live at The Drive after Bob took over as manager. Ellen would no longer have been a full member of the staff team; she would have reverted to being the 'domestic', an ancillary worker. Although Ellen might well have established an important relationship with Paul and might have gained access to his room to help him to clean it up, she would have been working in isolation, without official recognition that it was her role to engage with and respond to Paul. In Bob's scheme of things, domestic workers did not work with residents; they did the cleaning. She would certainly not have been expected to report back on this piece of work; she would not have had access to residents' files and would not have contributed to their care notes; she would not have attended staff or handover meetings and been able to offer her insight; she would not have been in a position to discuss with Paul and help him to think about any decisions to do with the decoration and furnishing of his room, or to do with food and mealtimes. If she had 'reported' the evidence of drugs and alcohol in the room, she would not have been consulted on what action should be taken, and Bob might well have decided to get rid of Paul. If she had not 'reported' the evidence, and if Bob had found out that she had known, she might have been disciplined. (He would probably have welcomed the chance of 'easing her out'!) Even if, under this new regime, Ellen had managed to clean the room and had given Paul some useful support at the same time, he would have experienced her involvement with him not as a manifestation of the Home as a whole, but as the individual work of perhaps the one person who seemed to care and who could actually help him in some practical way. Under Bob's management, Ellen's readiness to engage and respond would have been unrepresentative and at odds with the culture of the Home. And now suppose that Ellen, disheartened by the downgrading of her job by her loss of authority and satisfaction, decided to leave? What chance would Paul then have had?

RESIDENTS' NEEDS CANNOT BE NEATLY SEPARATED

Individuals enter residential care not as a collection of neatly separated problems but as whole people with a range of needs which, if their assessment is accurate, can be met by living in a Home. All residents bring with them their talents; they bring strengths as well as weaknesses, enthusiasm as well as apathy – a fact that is ignored in highly institutionalised settings where people 'become' the most prominent of their disabilities, illnesses or frailties. In some nursing Homes people enter care carrying their medical or quasi-medical 'definition' with them and are thereafter referred to as 'a stroke', 'a diabetic', 'an epileptic' or 'an amputee'. It is quite common now to hear 'an Alzheimer's' used to describe any older person who appears to have some sort of dementia – in the same inaccurate and catch-all way as 'confused', 'senile dementia', even 'gaga' and 'babies' were formerly used. In an unconscious attempt to reduce the anxiety associated with working closely with a resident – with facing the very personal and frightening experience of getting to know the person who is living with this disability or that frailty – staff groups, Homes and organisations lump people together in categories of special need and fit them into 'units' of residential provision. Staff can then become relatively uninvolved with the whole person, and work only with whatever assessed problem that person has. In many Homes incontinence serves as a very important prop in these defences against the anxiety engendered by involvement with the person. Older and disabled people are kept incontinent because, unpleasant as the task of dealing with the results is, people's incontinence becomes their principle feature. It is time-consuming, repetitive and fruitless to take people to the toilet – after they have wet or messed themselves – to wipe them, wash them, 'pad them up' and then take them back to sit and wait for the next round; but such work defines and delineates a merely functional relationship in which the deeply personal implications of losing control of one's body in this most undignified way are avoided. Eventually most residents accept their 'incontinent' role.

Mr Brown (p. 91), at Norwood House, could have become and been known as his 'problem' – a 'wanderer'. This is why staff at the Home were reluctant to use the word for fear of isolating a bit of his behaviour as representative of the whole person. On the other hand, the assistant director readily spoke of residents, who had even once been 'missing' for just a few minutes, as 'wanderers' – an approach which enabled him to produce one-dimensional 'solutions' to what he regarded as simple 'problems'. If he could have locked 'wanderers' in, he would have done so.

In 'secure units' run by social services for young offenders, residents are often defined by their crime – 'This one's a TDA (taking and driving away), that one's a GBH (grievous bodily harm), and that one over there, he's in for rape and he's Section 53 (sentenced to detention under Section 53 of the *Children and Young Persons Act* 1933).' If there is any genuine intention to help such young people to grow up into, and to experience themselves as, whole people, it will be done slowly with an integrated team of whole, all-rounded, mature people working in a Home which provides an integrated experience of living – all aspects of living.

Residents, too, quickly begin to experience and define themselves as simply a sum of their disability, illness, crime, deprivation, delinquency or frailty. Homes which use this labelling and depersonalising as a way of dealing with the enormous anxiety of getting to know and work with the whole person are actively assisting the further disintegration of residents' lives. (Staff do not deliberately set out to do this; it is an unconscious defence against anxiety.)

Just as residents are represented to staff by their 'problem' or 'diagnosis', so staff are compartmentalised by residents and by each other into separate roles, functions, hierarchies and attitudes. Instead of the valuable differences between the various members of a team being available to residents as resources to draw on, their individual distinctiveness is experienced as divisive. Sexuality and race, culture and age come between staff, splitting them into good and bad, friends and enemies, familiar and alien.

CHOPPED UP CARE

To manage this complex whole without resorting to chopping it up into manageable little pieces begins to sound like an impossible task. The management task has been divided into its main elements in this book – meeting residents' needs by managing staff, buildings and equipment, and money – but when it is subdivided into further parts (such as staffing numbers and costs) we find that nothing can in fact be confined to the compartment in which we attempted to place it. Many organisations react to this problem by setting up separate 'divisions' and 'sections' (the words are important) to deal with separate aspects of residential care. (An unconscious defence such as this cannot be worked against while it is not known about.) So 'human resources' manage staffing; the 'training section' manage training and staff development; the 'finance section' manage money (often residents' money as well); the supplies contracts manager buys the food and cleaning materials on a three-year deal; the 'quality and resources' division manages standards of care; the 'maintenance section' (of another 'division' or 'directorate') get the drains cleared – but only after they have received an official order from the 'admin section'; 'environmental services' manage the gardens; and someone from 'design and display' (a section of the 'directorate of development') decides what curtains will be hung in the sitting room. Yet the declared aim of the organisation is to run residential services that are homely.

Generally, organisations cannot contemplate the glaring contradiction between their stated aims and the obvious results of their actions. When presented with the crude truth of the effects of chopping up management functions and responsibilities, and of ignoring repeated guidance about the importance of maintaining the Home managers' authority (Skinner 1992), senior managers assert that managers of Homes are not competent to cope with the demands of managing staffing, maintenance and finance. Yet, by keeping power in their own hands, they are left with Homes which have no clear leadership, no authority, no coherent philosophy and no sense of primary task. In hierarchical structures the Homes are outposts of the central organisation, and the people appointed to lead and manage them are used as mere ciphers in a chain of command. This was the sort of management approach which infuriated Rachel at Norwood House and made Thomas determined to look for another job after his responsibilities had been usurped in the local authority for which he had worked before going to The Limes. And it was a management approach which Janet felt she had been unwittingly drawn into, but was determined to change with Jeeva's help.

THERAPEUTIC WORK: BRINGING THE PARTS TOGETHER

As the director of care services for Hetherington Housing, Janet had to visit Homes quite frequently on official business. While she was there she would take the opportunity to talk with residents and with staff, and she tried to notice what was going on. If she saw things happening which clearly did not conform to the housing association's policy, she would usually take up the point directly with a member of staff and would later discuss it with Jeeva. Although she and Jeeva worked extremely well together, she found his attitude could seem almost evasive during discussions of what had appeared to her to be poor care practice. Jeeva said that some things were difficult to explain to an outsider who didn't understand the background. How, he asked, could outsiders expect to be able to comprehend the intricate and interlocking issues of life in a residential community when they had no experience of coping with them? Janet's observations and concerns as an outsider were none the less useful and relevant, and Jeeva listened to them and gave them much thought, but they also revealed the limitations of her understanding. The turning point, at which Janet decided that she must really understand what was going on, came one day when she witnessed an extraordinary scene in the sitting room of one of the Homes.

A member of staff was almost shouting at an old man sitting in a wheelchair, saying, 'No, I will not make you a cup of tea. I've told you a dozen times that you can make your own tea, and I'm fed up with repeating myself. The next time you ask me like that, I shan't even reply.' Janet noticed that the resident had one leg amputated at the knee. Looking crestfallen and humiliated, and with tears in his eyes, he propelled his wheelchair out of the sitting room. Janet was shocked. She tried to speak to the member of staff, who looked very flustered but said that she was sorry but she was unable to talk about it because she was too busy. Janet found the nursing team manager who said she was very busy too and it might be difficult to explain; why didn't she ask Jeeva about it? Janet could only conclude that they were avoiding discussing something they knew was wrong and were hoping that Jeeva would produce some excuses for them.

Janet spoke to Jeeva as soon as possible: 'If a resident wants a cup of tea made at any time, he should be able to have one. Our policies are quite clear and we even write in our brochures that residents can ask for and get drinks whenever they want them. And, in any case, no member of staff should speak to a resident like that. I think she should be disciplined.' Jeeva said that he didn't think the scene was at all extraordinary. Knowing the resident and the member of staff, he wasn't worried by what Janet had heard and seen, although he was concerned that what was going on might easily (and understandably) have been misinterpreted by any outsider. It seemed to Janet that Jeeva's response was more to do with how things looked than with residents' well-being, and yet she knew that was not how he worked.

Jeeva knew that Janet needed to understand and, warning her that they would need at least an hour to talk, he tried to explain. The member of staff, Hyacinth, was a well-experienced senior worker. She had been at the Home for several years and had participated in the progressive developments which had taken place since Jeeva had been involved. At first, like many other members of staff, she had been reluctant to change well-worn patterns of work and attitudes which came from her training and long experience as a nurse in a hospital. However, she had stuck with the discussions, arguing her case strongly, but gradually bringing about her own deep changes in her whole approach to and philosophy about the work. Initially Hyacinth appeared to be quite a rigid person but, once he got to know her, Jeeva soon found that she was very different. They had built a mutual respect which was based on each of them holding apparently conflicting opinions and being comfortable talking with each other about them. Once Hyacinth realised that Jeeva was not a manager who, like so many she had known, was going to tell her what to think, she could afford to relax her tight hold on the strict nursing procedures and practices, adherence to which had enabled her to achieve her position as a ward sister in the hospital. Jeeva also knew that her 75-year-old father was very ill and she was under considerable strain looking after him at home. In Jeeva's view, it was people like Hyacinth who were at the centre of the continuing development of good practice at the Home. Yet his relaxed view that the incident was not something to worry about was not based solely on his high opinion of Hyacinth's character and work; nor was he making excuses for her because of her stressful personal commitments. Jeeva knew a lot about the resident involved. For the last six months, he and the staff had been meeting regularly to discuss how best to work with him.

Mr Scott had come to the Home from hospital after having his leg amputated at the knee. He had diabetes and had lived at home before going into hospital. His wife, who had looked after him, had died two years previously. They had no children. After his wife's death, Mr Scott had been given a succession of daily home helps, all of whom had found him rude, unreasonable and demanding. In some instances, he had told the home care manager that he didn't want them to come back. In others, the home helps themselves refused to return to his flat because of his behaviour.

Mr Scott had treated his wife in much the same way, and although home care had been offered before she died, he wouldn't allow anyone to do work that he thought his wife should do. As a young soldier, he had survived three years in a Japanese prisoner of war camp and came back from this terrible experience a changed man. He trusted no one and disliked 'foreigners'.

When Mr Scott came from hospital to see the nursing Home, he showed no enthusiasm but said that he didn't care where he went so long as he had a room, a bed and three meals a day. He did not wish to see other Homes and would go where he was 'put'. He was given every chance to find out about the Home and the staff told him all about it, but he was steadfastly uninterested.

Staff from the Home and the care manager who was placing Mr Scott attempted to get him involved in making a care plan, but he simply agreed to everything which was suggested and said that he didn't care anyway, because his 'life was over'. The staff team knew that they were taking on a difficult task. Mr Scott had only recently lost his leg, and two years previously his wife had died after waiting on him hand and foot for most of their lives together. He was a very unhappy person, and seemed a little mad with his dislike of everything and everyone around him.

During his first few months at the Home, the staff team took great care in their work with him. He was indeed rude, demanding and unapproachable, but Hyacinth in particular was making some headway with him. Although she had, long ago, dropped much of her brisk, detached nursing style with most residents, she found that Mr Scott responded best to precisely that style. She became the ward sister again in his presence and he accepted her care and did as he was told when she behaved like that. He relaxed into the institutional care and relationships which were being provided specially for him; but this was just the first part of the staff team's plan for working with him. Hyacinth would sometimes find him near to tears and, if no one else was around, he would say something – at first about the amputation, then about his wife, and later he even mentioned the camp. Hyacinth knew both that she was making remarkable progress and that there would be difficult times to come. Mr Scott had taken to holding her hand fleetingly in the only friendly touch that he had given or received for many years, before he and Hyacinth reverted to the clear and well-defined nurse/patient mode of relating which he found easiest to cope with.

Mr Scott was prey to many emotional and physical problems, some of which he fought against and attempted to hide by his unremitting rudeness and hostility. Whether much of it – since his wartime experiences – was of his own doing or not, Mr Scott had lived a horribly unhappy life; but since he had first come to the Home, one of his major problems had been very evident to all – to staff, to other residents, even sometimes to visitors. Mr Scott was a racist. He was White and he was convinced that he hated Black people. He hated women too. Hyacinth was a Black woman.

Before he ever said anything, most of the staff – White and Black – knew that Mr Scott had these problems, but he had come to a Home and a group of staff who were prepared for him, and were strong enough to work with a man like him.

Decisions about admissions to this Home were made by the nursing team manager in consultation with the rest of the team and with Jeeva. They had made a decision to accept and work with Mr Scott and his pernicious behaviour. They knew what they were taking on and felt that they could do a good job.

Unlike many other places, this Home did not have an underlying culture in which Mr Scott's blatant racism could fester and spread. Indeed the place was overtly multiracial and multicultural. Though partly an expression of his terrible sense of loss, Mr Scott's determined lack of interest in the Home was probably his way of blocking out the strong (and, to him, challenging) message given during his visit to the building. The whole place could hardly have failed to have an impact: its decoration and furnishing, the pictures and photographs, the staff, the food, the other residents, the music, the activities, the conversation, the ways people related to each other and their sense of individual and collective authority and purpose. In all its variety, the message was strong and coherent. The nursing team manager thought it was significant that Mr Scott had chosen to ignore – and, thereby, to deny – the message, rather than actively rejecting the Home and asking to see somewhere else. It was almost as if he wanted to come to a place where this poisonous flaw in his personality might be excised. Probably without being conscious of it, and certainly without being able to admit it, he was in some way aware that this Home was his only hope of regaining the self-respect which had been wrenched out of him in the camp so long ago.

Neither residents nor staff gave the slightest encouragement to Mr Scott's racism. His previous experience led him to assume that the White staff and residents would agree with his racist sentiments, even if they 'hadn't got the guts to come out with it'. (Before he went into hospital, the home care manager had tried to find him White home helps because he said he wouldn't accept Black ones.) But he was isolated and cold-shouldered when he behaved badly, though some residents and staff actually pitied his plight. Like her, some of Hyacinth's colleagues were concerned for him and were professionally interested in the pathology of his 'condition'. Most of the Black staff had already seen such rabid racism in many work and social situations, but had never before been in an environment that enabled them to work with someone who had 'got it'. They felt that they were dealing with a sort of sickness with which they could quite objectively help the 'sufferer', rather than simply have to cope with its corrosive results.

Although Hyacinth was at the centre of implementing a care plan for Mr Scott, she was not, of course, the only member of staff who worked with him. For the first few months of his stay the number of people who gave him direct care was kept to a minimum. Consistency was seen to be vital for Mr Scott, even more than it was for other residents. At first, the plan was to give him all the physical care which he wanted and needed, and to provide it in a detached and 'clinical' way which protected both staff and Mr Scott from the threat of personal relationships. (With Jeeva's consultative help, staff were well aware that almost exactly the same actions could result from unconscious defences against anxiety. They were consciously using this mode of care to enable Mr Scott to accept help and to establish an initial way of relating to staff which was rather mechanistic and relatively unthreatening.) As the more personal relationship with Hyacinth emerged, she introduced ways in which Mr Scott could do more for himself. He began to transfer himself from his wheelchair to his bed, and to dress himself – at first, only 'for' Hyacinth, but gradually he began to help himself more when others worked with him. However, moments of personal engagement when he spoke of his feelings (rather than acting them out) occurred only with Hyacinth and were a long time coming.

When Mr Scott found that he was trusting and confiding in Hyacinth, he 'defended' his deeply ingrained racism by arguing that she was different – different from all the other Black people he had encountered (but whom he had never got to know). Hyacinth was a nurse who, he told himself, had the misfortune to be Black, but who had all the qualities which he attributed to a good White nurse. Of course, Hyacinth had made no compromises with her ethnicity and culture. She knew that to give Mr Scott an inch by pandering to this defensive delusion that he could 'overlook' her colour would in fact destroy his flickering trust and dump him back at square one. In any case, however seductive, this was a collusion which she had encountered many times before in nursing and would never contemplate entering into.

This work with Mr Scott was desperately difficult for all concerned. There was no smooth progress. The advances which were made in the privacy of his room appeared to be quickly undone in the more public areas of the Home, where he would curse and insult staff, and order them about; ignore Black residents and try to enlist the allegiance of White residents; refuse and disparage food which was 'not English'. Under such an onslaught of hatred most other Homes would have given up, but although Mr Scott's behaviour was hurtful and disturbing, the self-confidence woven into the resilient fabric of life and work at this Home enabled staff to withstand these attacks. Furthermore, this Home had a clear therapeutic plan. The strength came from the combination and inter-relatedness of all aspects of the Home in accomplishing its primary task. No part of the Home was made vulnerable by being disconnected from the whole.

The incident which had worried Janet so much, and which Jeeva was now attempting to put into this complicated context, occurred about six months after Mr Scott had come to the Home. By now he was doing quite a lot for himself and, in spite of major rows as he and Hyacinth established a closer relationship, he had confided in her consistently, and had begun to accept and be more respectful to other staff as well. All members of the team had gradually changed their way of responding to his racist and sexist attacks. Instead of ignoring them, they simply withdrew from caring for him when he made them. Their line was, 'I will not put up with that sort of talk, Mr Scott. If you want my help, you will have to treat me with the same respect which I give you. I will come back in a few minutes to see if I can carry on with what I was doing for you.' This entailed taking some risks because Mr Scott was sometimes intent on 'teaching them a lesson'. Of course, they took care not to leave him suspended on a bath hoist (though occasionally such fantasies did come to mind!), but he was quite capable of leaving the wash-basin to overflow and flooding his room in retribution for being abandoned. Members of the team also emphasised to Mr Scott that they worked as a team, so that he could not pretend that insulting and abusive behaviour to one worker would be ignored when he was with someone he got on with better. They would directly confront him with his bad behaviour to a colleague, saying that they worked with them and they were friends so they were not going to go along with his upsetting them. The new approach had paid off: Mr Scott was enjoying his new-found capacity for ordinary courtesy, and he got a lot of acknowledgement from Hyacinth for his efforts. 'Under that gruff exterior beats a warm, good heart. A lamb in wolf's clothing – you old devil,' she would say putting an arm round him. But outside the privacy of his room, the bathroom or lavatory, Mr Scott continued to disgrace himself. It seemed as if he felt he had to keep up appearances. If he let down his aggressive guard in public, who knows what might happen?

When he came into the Home he had brought nothing with him, but the nursing team manager had asked the care manager who placed him to collect from his flat all the things which she thought could be of use or value to him later. Mr Scott had told the care manager, 'Chuck it all away. I don't want any of it. My life's over anyway. Just bring my telly.' Although officially she should have carried out his instructions, she decided not to. She collected a few boxes of photographs and small bits and pieces, an electric kettle, a radio, some ornaments and two items of furniture – a chair and a glass-fronted cabinet. As Mr Scott began to settle down and to talk about his life, Hyacinth had let him know that some things had been kept from his flat and it hadn't all been dumped as he had asked. After a few days had passed and his initial tirade – against 'that bitch' (the care manager), who hadn't done what she said she would do ('you can't trust anyone') – had died down, Mr Scott asked Hyacinth about his stuff. Then they began rearranging his room, looking at the photos, and setting out the ornaments. Of course, many of the things had very sad and painful memories for him, and he didn't yet want to look at all of the photographs or to take out some of his other possessions; but Hyacinth had insisted on putting out the kettle, teapot and cups and saucers. She found a tray and a low table to put them on. Mr Scott did like his tea but he had not made himself tea since he was first married. Hyacinth said it was about time he did. 'I've been making you tea for six months now, and I think that's enough. It's high time you made me a cup. I'll get you tea bags, milk and sweeteners, and we'll do the washing up for you – only to begin with, mind you.'

It was a couple of days after that conversation that Janet had heard Hyacinth 'shouting' at Mr Scott in the sitting room. She had set out all the tea-making things and had given him careful instructions, but Mr Scott had steadfastly refused to make himself tea. It was a matter of principle for both sides. This was a benchmark for Mr Scott; if he started making himself tea, he would have lost a principle which had propped up his horrible life for the last fifty years. He was struggling not to let go of it, but neither Hyacinth nor any other member of staff would now make him tea. Of course, he had the drinks which were provided at the usual times and as much as he wanted. He knew that other residents could get drinks in between times – as the Home's brochure promised, they only had to ask. But Mr Scott's increasingly rude demands for tea were now being refused. The battle had gone on for two days. His language became more extreme and he seemed to be reverting to unleashing all the bigoted bile that had characterised his first few months in the Home. Hyacinth was more upset by not being able to make him a drink than she was by his disgusting behaviour. For once, she was doubting her own resolve. She was in tears with her colleagues, who were not tempted to give in. Steeling herself, Hyacinth rehearsed her response to Mr Scott's next demand . . . and that's what Janet heard: 'No, I will not make you a cup of tea. I've told you a dozen times that you can make your own tea, and I'm fed up with repeating myself. The next time you ask me like that, I shan't even reply.'

When Hyacinth knocked on Mr Scott's door half an hour later, she got no answer. She was desperately worried, and, fearful of what she would find, she went in without his permission. He was sitting in his wheelchair by the low table, on which there was still a full cup of tea. His cheeks were wet with tears. He held out his hand to Hyacinth, as he had done on previous occasions when he had confided in her. She took his hand, and putting her other arm around his shoulders, she kissed him on the top of his head, and then, without a word, left the room in a hurry to find a colleague who could sit with her.

Had Janet seen Hyacinth enter Mr Scott's room without his permission and invade his personal space by kissing him, she would have been even more concerned about a member of staff who was working outside clearly prescribed, and universally accepted, codes of good practice.

In a Home pursuing a therapeutic task, staff had to take risks. The rules and procedures to which Janet attached so much importance were not invented for this sort of work. They were 'put in place' by people who had either never done it themselves or, if they had, they had forgotten what it felt like to engage their whole selves in this way. The carefully planned and coordinated work with Mr Scott attained a level of sophistication, courage and commitment far beyond what any outsider could imagine would ever be achieved in a nursing or residential care Home. Yet, with Jeeva's encouragement and wise counsel, it was the sort of work to which this Home was aspiring, and the rehabilitation of Mr Scott was a major milestone in its development.

Gripped by this story and feeling humbled by it, Janet felt like rushing back to the Home, finding Hyacinth and apologising to her for so misreading the situation. Yet, however enthralled she was by the work which Jeeva had described, she knew that she was still a long way from understanding it, and that she must find a way to learn.

Following this turning point, Janet's programme of more extended, 'out of hours' visits to the Homes coincided with a succession of problems caused by the complex contracting and subcontracting of services between her housing association, two community health services trusts and a local authority maintenance department. She had been in the Homes when key staff had been withdrawn to work elsewhere; when 'bank' staff had been drafted in at short notice to fill gaps; when cooks didn't turn up; and when urgent maintenance was left undone for weeks on end. With her growing understanding of the complex social ecology of residential and nursing care, she had realised how vulnerable it was to the total environment within which it must struggle to survive. Having witnessed the effects of these administrative and management failures, she was determined to sort them out, but found, as Jeeva had done on countless occasions, that she could get nowhere with the unaccountable organisations which were notionally 'responsible' but which left the Homes' staff to pick up the pieces and try to sustain their therapeutic work.

Janet's anger at seeing for herself the appalling results of these shambolic – but very expensive – contracts was welcome to Jeeva, who agreed that fundamental changes in organisation and management were essential; but Jeeva was also worried that the enormous effort involved in regaining full management of the Homes could be wasted, especially if the housing association took direct control and then simply replicated the same fundamental errors. These Homes had to be managed from inside, not by an ignorant and bureaucratic central organisation which, in its current state of awareness and development, would again impose management on the Homes with a book of procedures in one hand and a megaphone in the other.

THE SURVIVAL OF A THERAPEUTIC ECOLOGY IN A POOR ENVIRONMENT

Considering the very unsuitable arrangements for staffing, maintenance and finance, the progress of the Homes which Jeeva managed was surprising and remarkable. The nursing team managers and the staff in the two nursing Homes had made good progress in spite of these arrangements. Sometimes a Home might function well for several months without major clashes occurring with any of the hotchpotch of managers and administrators on whom it was dependent for supplies, maintenance, staffing and finance. During the first six months of Mr Scott's stay, there was a relatively quiet relationship between the Home and all the organisations involved. This allowed the staff to take charge of their work, and allowed it to progress without interference. Yet, as the time to renegotiate the care, 'hotel' and maintenance contracts grew closer, the anxiety of the negotiations began to intrude. So it was at this time (nearing the end of the financial year) when the community health care trust began to make savings in staff time. They simply stopped providing sufficient staff and moved experienced staff to fill gaps elsewhere. On the occasions when the staffing levels fell below the minimum allowed by registration, the trust drafted in hourly paid 'bank' staff, most of whom did not know the residents but had the advantage – to the trust – of costing much less than permanent staff to employ.

Although Hyacinth would have refused to go, like some of her colleagues, she could have been asked to move to another Home which was temporarily short of experienced and trained senior staff. Of course, the effects on her and on Mr Scott would have been disastrous. But when another worker of the same importance in the Home did move in these circumstances, there were immediate detrimental effects on all residents and staff, not just to the people with whom she had direct contact.

If the nursing team manager had not, in the first place, taken Mr Scott on, but if he had been placed in the Home against the better judgement of the manager, the placement would have failed within days. If the Home had not had access to Jeeva in a consultative capacity but had had contact with the responsible organisation (the housing association) only in a more conventional managerial relationship (controlling and monitoring), the staff team would not have had the opportunities for reviewing, reflective thinking and planning which were vital for the level of work they were doing with Mr Scott. If the staff had not taken control of their own rotas, ways of communicating, food, furniture and budgets, they could not have worked with Mr Scott in the ways they did. But *officially* they did not have this degree of control. Like many other Homes in similar situations, struggling to create a therapeutic ecology, a relatively chaotic wider environment actually suited their purposes better than a more rigid, organised and imposing governing organisation. Jeeva was worried that the housing association, as an organisation, was no more suitable to manage the staffing and the 'hotel' services than were the health service trusts. At least with the present arrangements, for most of the year there was a laxity about money and staffing which enabled him, the nursing team manager and the staff to create their own disciplined organisation to attend to the primary task.

The job of the responsible organisation is to create a wider organisational environment within which the self-managing, self-directed and, in many ways, self-sufficient social ecology of each Home can become established and flourish. This relationship parallels the one which the Home has with residents – creating an environment within which residents can be as independent and self-sufficient as possible (and as they wish). Of course, wider organisations which do create such an environment, which are reliable in their supply of all the resources necessary for the sustenance of a therapeutic ecology, and which are able to provide support and consultation in the way in which Jeeva provided it, are the organisations which are fit to run residential and nursing care.

Part IV

Outside influences

INSIDE/OUTSIDE

In order to manage residential care well – from the outside – we have to give up the notions of controlling and directing which are currently so central to most outside managers' philosophies. The life of a residential Home – what we have described as the therapeutic ecology – is essentially self-directed and self-regulating. There is no true life in a Home which does not itself change and evolve with the lives of the people who live and work there. The capacity to change is dependent on some aspects of life remaining constant but when consistency and regularity seem to prevail, disruption – joyful or painful – will be just around the corner. Using a wide range of skills and techniques, the care manager (the 'inside' manager) and the care team participate in (are part of) this ever-changing ecology of care. They are highly influential; they lead; they steer and guide; they hold and contain; they foster and encourage ... they manage, but they cannot direct and control, and they should not attempt to – and nor should the 'outside' manager.

The ecology of the Home exists within a larger environment – the organisation which runs the Home. That organisation is itself part of a larger social, political and economic environment. The 'environment' in this sense is not controllable, although it is populated by people who are attempting to bring it under control. If they can see and understand more of the whole picture, if they can know that they are a part of – participants in – this environment, they will then be in a position to influence and lead and to make their difference.

Residential Homes should be distinct, but not isolated units of organisation. Other than those small private Homes which have an owner/manager, Homes are usually a part of and 'managed' by a larger organisation, whether it is a private care company, a local authority, a charity or a housing association. The 'inside' view, from the Home outwards, is often hostile to the organisation which runs the Home by attempting to 'incorporate' it. ('Incorporation' in this sense is a combination of aggressive intervention and swallowing up. Homes become 'colonies' of the powerful outside organisation; indeed, the word 'colony' was used to describe large residential institutions.) The 'outside' view is frequently hostile both to the Home and to the very idea of residential care (see p. 67). There is a widespread and destructive antagonism between inside and outside.

Inside/outside antagonism was not part of the management culture of The Limes (Chapter 3) because its owner/manager Noreen had always worked in the Home; and after she had brought Thomas in as manager, she soon trusted him enough to let him take over the full management responsibilities. Though she remained very much involved, she did not interfere. However, even without an external management organisation, there was nevertheless a strong element of antagonism in her relationships with several outside bodies, notably with the inspection unit. She experienced them as ignorant, interfering and dictatorial busybodies. Noreen reacted badly to them and to any other powerful outside organisation which had the temerity to tell her how to run The Limes. It was only because of the sensible personal intervention of the chief inspector, and, later, because of Thomas's skilful and relaxed negotiation, that the Home and the inspection team did not become locked in battle over relatively trivial issues. Yet in her own way Noreen was an excellent manager, committed to the residents, fighting for their rights and welfare. This vehemence about the work itself made it difficult for outsiders to negotiate with her about a different way of working. She liked residents and staff who were 'difficult' and different, and she encouraged people to stand up for themselves and for what they believed in. The Limes would have been a very different place if it had been run by a local authority or housing association.

However, as we have seen, the outside organisation's insistent demand for conformity (with all its stultifying consequences) is sometimes resisted – though at a price. We have examples of Homes, their managers and staff who had managed to be different and to stand out against a tide of conformist mediocrity. Both Norwood House (Chapter 4) and the Homes which Jeeva managed (Chapter 5) were very different from the other Homes in the rest of their organisations. As a result, they had got a name (from outside) for being 'dangerous' or 'difficult', and the outside managers who worked with these staff groups and fostered the Homes' independent, self-directed stance were, in their turn, also seen to be difficult.

The dominant, management view of residential care as an area of operations which must be controlled by outside organisations is the one formed and circulated by outside managers. It is unfortunate that the same view is often grudgingly accepted by insiders – managers, staff and residents – who resent it, kick against it and complain about it, but do not set out to take control themselves and change it. The alternative view, consistently promoted in this book – that residential Homes can best be managed from inside, while being supported from outside – is, as yet, not widely understood and is rarely put into practice. This simple switch of direction in management is the key to providing good care. So many Homes which have been provided with all the necessary resources (except suitable management) have failed because organisations tried to manage them from outside.

The prevailing flow of management communication and influence runs counter to the direction which everyone agrees is right for client/ worker relationships. The worker's efforts should all lead the client towards self-sufficiency and self-direction. Although there are clearly times when the client must be supported through a state of dependency, and situations when some of the support must remain, at no time should the care worker 'take over' areas – however small – in which clients may take responsibility and exert control for themselves. Clearly, the model of organisation required to manage face-to-face care work must be built on a thorough comprehension of the nature of the care relationship itself, as has already been described in Chapter 6.

PRINCIPLES/PRACTICE

The growth of 'outsiders' in relation to residential care has been fuelled by organisations' addiction to the production of policy and procedure. We have seen how repeatedly setting out what staff in the organisation are going to do (policy) and how they are going to do it (procedure) can effectively protect senior figures in organisations from the charge of not doing it. 'Our policy is clear and we have issued procedures to all staff for its implementation,' they say, with the implication that, 'It is their fault if it isn't done, not ours.'

Policies and procedures connect the much more important principles and practice. It is the job of management within Homes to create policy and procedure (where necessary) in order to put principles into practice. Outside organisations have removed this connection and expend much time and energy on producing policy and procedure for the Homes which is then foisted on residential staff. They would be much more

properly engaged on supporting and resourcing Homes, and on producing policy at an organisational level which enables the Homes to
achieve their primary tasks.

In this last part of the book, we will examine ways in which 'outsiders' currently perform and recommend ways in which they could
contribute to achieving the primary task in Homes, rather than hindering
it.

Chapter 13

Feet of clay, seats of power, ivory towers – and egg mayonnaise on the keyboard

I'm the king of the castle . . .

Different worlds – The headquarters culture – Using boundaries creatively

DIFFERENT WORLDS

As well as being the most numerous and the most costly, residential Homes are the most distinct, clearly defined units of social care provision. (This combination of circumstances has made Homes the easiest parts of social services for local authorities to discard.) The organisations which provide residential care are not distinct entities; they are comparatively amorphous assemblages of various functions, though it may appear that their 'divisions', 'departments' and 'sections' are highly differentiated and clearly separated. When you go to the offices of the larger organisations, you will find many different collections of staff engaged on many different tasks. However much 're-engineering' has taken place, however fashionably 'delayered' or 'multiskilled' these organisations have become, they are still bureaucracies. The people in these office buildings plan, administrate and manage; they do not 'do'. Within the Homes, most of the workforce do; and, in addition, the residents live there. No one lives at the headquarters of the organisations. These are very different worlds.

Since 1961, when Erving Goffman's *Asylums* was first published, hundreds of thousands of students have readily absorbed a 'pop' critique of residential institutions. In addition to the widespread disdain of and long-held prejudices about residential Homes (see Chapter 7, p. 72), all those who have heard of 'institutionalisation' (but probably never actually read Goffman's wonderful book) have perpetuated a pseudo-sociological certainty about the iniquities of any form of residential care. They all suppose that they know what is wrong with residential Homes and how they would put it right. Generally these outsiders do not examine their own workplaces and their own unconscious institutionalisation. Lacking self-awareness in these areas and projecting fault on to those who are giving care, they are ill prepared for their dealings with residential Homes and approach them with a hostile attitude.

THE HEADQUARTERS CULTURE

When Jeeva first joined Hetherington Housing, he expected to find a much less bureaucratic and institutionalised, and much more self-aware and self-critical organisation than the local authority he had just left. He was surprised to find there was little difference.

The headquarters building where Jeeva worked was new. At the front it had high iron railings and large double gates, opened by remote control from the reception office. There was room for about eight VIP cars. The front door was guarded by closed circuit television cameras and an entry phone. From the outside the building looked grand – fortified – defended against the outside. People who worked in it had coded plastic cards which unlocked its doors, but tenants of the housing association came to this building as supplicants to a superior power. Once inside, tenants were politely asked to wait while a housing officer was called to come and see them. They would then meet in a room off the entrance hall, where they were placed in front of desks at which each 'customer services' officer sat consulting a computer screen, while having immediate access to a panic button concealed under the desk so that help could be summoned if a tenant got nasty. Tenants never went through the door which led into the main office area: they themselves were not the main business of the building. As with residential Homes, this building and the ways in which it was used said a lot. It quickly and clearly established a hierarchy of power, privilege and status in which everyone was effortlessly guided to her or his allotted place. Jeeva was accustomed to looking at every Home from the point of view of the resident or visiting relative, and he was amazed that the architects and planners had not been more sensitive in their design of this new headquarters building.

In many other ways, though, the building was well designed: light, airy and not too noisy. Jeeva's workspace was in a large open-plan area on the second floor where he worked in a small group with other residential care managers and administrators. Janet's office was on the ground floor near the chief executive's.

It took Jeeva some time to get to know the building and the different sections and all the people he had to work with in those sections. Although he spent much of his time out of the office and in the Homes, he began to observe – and to be fascinated by – the behaviour of the people around him in the headquarters building.

In a Home Jeeva instinctively noticed what would seem tiny and insignificant things to less experienced visitors; Jeeva knew that, on the contrary, they were important. How someone dressed, what people called each other, who made the tea and who cleared up were all important details to note in any residential Home. In the head office some of his colleagues were inclined to scorn any significance being attributed to such 'trivia', and other more senior managers would attempt to control the details of personal behaviour by instituting rules such as a 'dress code'. But because Jeeva had previously been a residential worker and manager, he was extra conscious of how *he* was now behaving, and he was worried about the gap which might open up between the way he and other people behaved in the head office, and the standards of behaviour he was expecting from staff in residential Homes. He not only felt that it would be dishonest to expect higher standards of people who were working under very much greater pressures, but he also knew that without attaining high standards themselves, and facing the personal challenges involved in doing so, any efforts by head office staff to influence changes in the Homes would be ineffectual and even counterproductive.

Staff at the head office brought items of personal significance to work and set them out on their desks or in their individual offices. Some were clearly chosen mainly to give a message to other people, and some were very much for themselves. Jeeva was moved by Janet's attempts to make her office personal and to express something about herself and her life. To him, the framed pictures of her children and partner, her son's paintings, and the photographs of her as a young woman doing her voluntary service overseas in Africa, were very genuine, and not a carefully selected exhibition designed more to impress than to give her pleasure. In some other senior managers' offices, such personal pictures looked to him more like trophies, very like the 'happy family' photographs of politicians who seem to be 'protesting too much' when they parade their personal lives to try to win popular approval.

As he did in residential care, Jeeva found one of the most revealing areas of behaviour was the way in which people 'catered' for themselves – making drinks and food, and how they consumed them. One of the hallmarks of good residential work is the extent to which staff share everyday living experience with residents, and easily and naturally make such events as mealtimes and coffee breaks convivial social occasions. Most of his colleagues at the headquarters building would find such sociability very threatening. Of course, there was not the same necessity for sharing such events; it was certainly not a regular part of anyone's job to eat or have coffee together. However, the ways in which so many of these head office staff behaved revealed such a low level of self-awareness that they would find it impossible to understand what the more forward-looking Homes were asking of them in the way of support and good administration.

How would some of them make sense of Jeeva's insistence that when staff ate with residents they should not pay for their meals because it was an important part of their job? Jeeva was not optimistic that his arguments would persuade the man in the finance section who brought in his elaborate packed lunch each day, and at precisely 12.30 p.m. cleared his desk and set out the same carefully wrapped sandwiches, piece of fruit, crisps, cake, yoghurt and carton of drink. At 1 p.m. he had finished, and after packing away the plastic boxes and wiping the desk meticulously, he resumed his work. During his half-hour lunch break, he was not to be disturbed – certainly not in order to discuss 'free lunches' for residential workers. As he ate he read a computer magazine propped on the desk in front of him. No one had ever been offered so much as a crisp.

Although there were a few who bought sandwiches for each other, shared food and enjoyed being together, most people made their own individual arrangements. Jeeva was fascinated by the people who kept biscuits in their desk drawers but rarely offered them to anyone else; by their special jars of coffee which they locked away; and by the very ways people consumed their food and drink. There were several greedy biscuit noshers – nibbling one after the other, scrunching very fast, until the plate was cleared. If he found himself in a meeting with one of these ultra-anxious munchers, he had to make a conscious effort not to stare at the biscuit-devouring performance. The fancy ground-coffee fusspots contrasted with the slapdash – don't wait for the kettle to boil – shake in sugar and granules – slop in the milk – give it a quick stir and throw the teaspoon in the sink – instants. In the communal give-and-take of residential care such behaviour becomes an issue and will be discussed.

Jeeva was embarrassed to join the senior staff who sent out for smart sandwich lunches at the drop of a hat and made sure that the underling who actually walked round to the new sandwich joint bought them their favourite chocolate biscuits as well – all on the firm, of course. He was repelled by the sight of young men sitting at their desks ploughing their way through a great big cardboard plateful of microwaved 'dinner' with not a glance or word, their noses, when not close to the plate to aid the accuracy of the rhythmic shovelling, stuck in the sports pages of a newspaper or in a car magazine. Again, no one in the office had to face the issues raised by their 'personal' behaviour, and would be unlikely to understand that staff in a good residential Home do have to face these issues every hour of every day.

So much was revealed in other related areas of behaviour as well, such as whether people cleared up after themselves or not. Some left the lavatories dirty, or left mugs and other debris from their personal 'catering' all around their offices for the cleaners to come and clear up later. The conscientious team members tried to get the others to behave properly and keep things clean and tidy – but failed miserably and resorted to composing ever more desperate notices: 'Please leave this toilet as you would want to find it'; 'Please wash up and put away your mugs and teaspoons before leaving this kitchen' – all to no avail. These personal 'living' arrangements in the office lurched between 'everyone for themselves' at one extreme, and at the other the tea clubs and washing-up rotas. Sometimes there were long discussions in meetings which attempted to find ways of regulating behaviour without understanding the behaviour itself.

One of Jeeva's colleagues was a 'jacket on the back of the chair – I'm a hard worker – in the office before the chief executive – work late – out to impress' young manager. Another was a laid-back, 'seen it all before – going through the motions – as soon as I get another job, I'm out of here' cynic. One whom Jeeva found particularly aggravating was the 'personal phone calls – waiting in for the gas man – flu four times a year – it's not fair that I have to pay my own parking fines' half-timer paid at full-time rates. But equally annoying was the 'do as I'm told but hate every minute of it' dogsbody. Very few people had an inkling of what it would take for them to work as a team – together.

These office 'characters' were not much good at their work, and with too many of them an organisation grinds to a halt. Janet and her fellow directors found the organisational inertia exasperating. To some extent it was created – and it was certainly held in place – by this unofficial social system in which everyone indulged his or her own independent patterns of behaviour in spite of the repeated efforts (rules and guidelines) to try to get some 'corporate' code of conduct established. When the information technology section was faced with the week's fourth computer breakdown due to coffee, crumbs or egg mayonnaise in keyboards, the director of human resources issued the edict that henceforth staff would not be allowed to eat or drink at their desks. The director had forgotten that he himself nearly always ate his favourite egg mayonnaise sandwiches at his desk – if he wasn't eating even smarter sandwiches in the boardroom – and some of the 'bolshier' staff were quite happy to point this out to him when they refused to comply with the ban. The union was involved; there were several long meetings, a considerable disruption to regular work, and a lot of bad feeling before the director of human resources issued a further memo to all staff, asking them to be 'very careful' not to get crumbs or coffee (he didn't like to mention the egg mayonnaise) anywhere near their computers.

Jeeva spent more than half his working week in the Homes, so he was a somewhat detached observer of these office antics. He was troubled by his involvement, which felt like collusion particularly because he could see what was happening and knew he had a part in it, but felt unable to change it. He was also exasperated by the adverse effects on the running of the Homes. The organisation was too often incapable of responding promptly, clearly, consistently and helpfully to the most straightforward of requests. It was very difficult to get a director of human resources who issued directives about not eating at desks and was about to launch a 'dress code' (for residential staff as well as head office staff) to understand that changing staff practices in Homes required a lengthy process of discussion, increasing understanding and awareness, which would then enable staff themselves to make deep and long-lasting changes. The human resources department's approach to changing practice was to 'write a good procedure'.

The failure of the housing association to become a learning and developing organisation, and its entrenched lack of cooperative teamwork, were among the reasons why Janet had found it so difficult to alter her own approach to residential Homes. She was viewing them from outside through a very distorted lens. At first, instead of understanding the Homes from the inside, she both assumed that work attitudes and relationships there would be similar to those she found so aggravating in the headquarters organisation, and projected the unacknowledged faults on to the Homes. It was not until she got 'inside' the work of the residential staff that she was able to begin to see it all very differently, and to be much more optimistic about long-term changes.

Generally, outside managers and administrators, isolated in their ivory tower headquarters, are simply unfitted to understand the issues of residential work. They are in no position to manage effectively. Clinging on to control of the internal affairs of Homes, they have no appreciation of the significance of their behaviour at work, of their management decisions or the effects in the Homes themselves of that behaviour or those decisions.

USING BOUNDARIES CREATIVELY

Having gained awareness of their own behaviour in relation to Homes, to manage effectively, outside managers must recognise residential Homes as distinct entities. Each Home, run as a largely autonomous organisation, with its own primary task, its own team, its own buildings and equipment, and its own budget, must function within its own boundary. All that takes place within the Home's boundary, and all the transactions across it (between it and its environment) must be controlled from within the Home (see Chapter 6). Responsibility for the work and functions of the Home can be further subdivided by time (e.g. managing a shift), by place (e.g. managing a group living unit), by specific areas of work (e.g. managing training), and by areas of care with particular clients (e.g. keyworking and the sort of therapeutic attention which Ellen managed with Paul in Chapter 6, pp. 56–61).

Managers outside the residential Home, like Jeeva and Janet, can envisage their own management roles and boundaries in a similar way. This will help them to define and carry out their responsibilities. While boundaries are hazy and indistinct or are being arbitrarily shifted, Homes without a defined and well-founded identity will merge and disappear into an amorphous 'organisation' that is no more than an assemblage of widely different and constantly changing 'non-organisations'.

Lacking the control which they crave over their own spheres of responsibility, managers frequently resort to interfering in the smaller units which are not their direct responsibility. So widespread is this practice that it has been mistaken for good practice. In fact it is the most insidious corrosion of management, which leads to the disintegration of the necessary structure of an organisation. In social care work – and particularly in residential care – the corrosion spreads rapidly, and soon distorts the vital relationship between care worker and client.

There is a good deal of sensible modern management advice and theory (e.g. Drucker 1979) which demonstrates how important clarity of role and tasks is to a manager at any level. That is not to say that managers should not be multiskilled and entrepreneurial, but that they should always be clear about the purpose and boundaries of their own jobs and those of the people they manage. As soon as a manager starts doing the job of someone whom she or he manages, rather than helping that person to manage her or his own work properly, the boundary is broken and very soon other boundaries will be bent, twisted or obliterated. All boundaries touch many other boundaries; distort one, and others buckle under the pressure. Sometimes job descriptions of managers are an indication of this corruption. Three jobs – for example, a care manager of a Home, her service manager, and the service manager's manager – will be described as sharing large common areas of responsibilities and tasks, demonstrating that the organisation which employs them has no idea of the importance of defining management boundaries.

We have seen how a disciplined framework of responsibilities and integrated roles is essential in residential work. If staff do not know 'where they are' in relation to other staff – who's doing what and when – clients' needs and some clients' delinquencies can fall through the spaces between a poorly coordinated staff group. The same clear structures and boundaries, and a commitment to maintaining them, are no less essential in the organisations within which residential Homes are managed.

The mistake is to see a 'boundary' as a 'division' rather than a delineation of a relationship – as a separation rather than a meeting. The boundary is therefore attacked and defended, rather than negotiated and agreed. We have considered the corruption and breakdown of boundaries as they are broken and bent, but the positive use of boundaries is that they are defining points of communication – that transactions across boundaries are mutually agreed exchanges and transfers of responsibility. Each boundary is contingent on all the boundaries it shares. When conceived and used in this creative way, boundaries are therefore constantly on the move, but they move in conjunction with one another. Think of the boundaries between worker and client: as the client changes, the boundaries which she shares with the worker and with the wider ecology of the Home also change. Or consider the boundaries between individuals within a team of workers: as each moves into new responsibilities or takes on the keyworker task with a resident, every other team member's boundaries shift accordingly. Or the boundary shared between the care manager and the service manager: as the care manager moves into the area of budget management or decisions about admissions, so the service manager's boundaries move to accommodate the changes which they have worked on together.

We have analysed this inside/outside relationship between the Home (and its care manager and staff) and the organisation (and its managers and administrative staff). We have looked at how the relationship goes wrong – how it is often negative, hostile and unhelpful – and how it can be conducted creatively, productively and supportively. The key to effective management relationships is for all participants to know – and to agree – what their tasks and responsibilities are, and to be clear about their own roles in carrying them out.

The inside/outside confusion is not confined to managerial relationships, and it is further complicated by the jumbled profusion of the many other 'outside' bodies which relate to residential care, some of which we look at in the next two chapters.

Chapter 14

The policy élite

Little Jack Horner sat in a corner, eating his pudding and pie . . .

Beyond the management: the policy-makers – The political and economic abuses of residential care – Training and the policy élite – The civil service élite – The exclusiveness of club membership

BEYOND THE MANAGEMENT – THE POLICY MAKERS

In Chapter 13 we discussed the personnel of the organisations which run residential care and we referred to the managers and administrators who work in them as 'outsiders'. (It is ironic that residential workers often feel that it is they who are the outsiders – outside their organisations, and outside the standard, nine-to-five, Monday-to-Friday world of office work.) Yet the outside organisations previously described are only a part of the environment surrounding residential Homes. Beyond them lies the 'policy community' – and that is where the big decisions about residential care are taken and where the direction of policy is set. As we know, the working relationship between the outside organisation and the Home can be difficult, yet however strained and distant their communication may be, there is, at least, contact; but with the policy community, residential Homes have no contact (Figure 14.1).

The stories of managers in Part I described their work inside and outside Homes. We have followed the development of those managers and considered the contexts in which they work, but the whole of residential care – residents, relatives, staff, managers and the organisations running the Homes – exists within a wider political and policy context. Residential care is a major political and economic issue partly

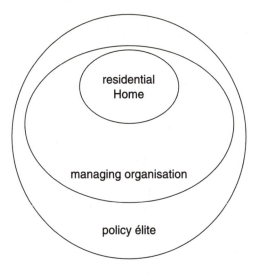

Figure 14.1

because it is a significant sector of local and national economies, and partly because it concerns or touches the lives and futures of most of the population in some way. Our arguments in this chapter are that, in spite of the vast resources which are consumed in generating legislation, policy, guidance, and grand planning for implementation, surprisingly little of direct use is produced, and, of that, even less is applied in practice to make a positive difference to people's lives in residential Homes. Although we have argued that the residential care of older people, for instance, is given insufficient resources and the needs of residents themselves are not taken seriously enough, there is no doubt that politicians, policy-makers and the public are indeed very concerned about the effects of the 'demographic time bomb' and the issues of paying for care in old age. In addition, there is deep public anxiety about what goes on in Homes. During an unprecedented period of investigation and scandal in residential child care, constant new legislation and guidance, a huge reduction in the overall number of children's Homes (but a very large increase in the number of privately run Homes and fostering agencies), and steeply rising costs for children living in care, the average quality of provision is now no better – and may be considerably worse – than it was.

There is constant, high-level (and expensive) activity as each public and political concern comes to the fore, but the *outcome* for clients of social care is minimal. Great savings could be made and transferred nearer to the point where care is provided. For every Kahan (1994), Warner (1992), Wagner (1988) and Avebury (1996) producing excellent, usable ideas and recommendations (though many of them remain unimplemented), there are several dozen other members of the policy élite who do scarcely more than talk and write to each other, and produce very little positive material. We will look at ways in which the overarching 'policy community' serves purposes unconnected with providing good services, and we will consider examples of the ways in which particular sections operate.

First let us recognise the corruption of power, money and status which has mired so many of the senior people who are members of this policy élite. Very high salaries are now being paid to the chief executives and heads of health and social services organisations, whether they are public, semi-public (health, housing and social care trusts), charitable or private. Salaries of £80,000 are not uncommon, but such levels of pay are defended by arguing that they are less than the equivalent managers would receive for similar responsibilities in most other areas of work. In addition, senior managers are given perks and bonuses of all sorts. They 'trade' in their supposed expertise and in return receive handsome 'consultancy' fees, even while they are employed. Their 'payoffs' when they leave a job are gross. Just like their counterparts in 'privatised' industries, utilities and services, they are quick to jump at money-making sell-offs, and 'management buy-outs' are on the increase. Only a small proportion of this graft and corruption is publicly revealed, but even when it is, the news is received with no great surprise.

In a recent example, the findings of the National Health Service (NHS) Executive and the House of Commons Public Accounts Committee that the boss of a health authority had 'failed to discharge his duty of care' did not stop him from becoming the head of the NHS Executive in another region, or later from becoming director of research at a university. The director of personnel in the same authority awarded large contracts to her husband's firm, and shortly before the closure of the authority she was promoted to make sure that she received a higher redundancy package. Such dubious deals did not prevent her from getting consultancy work from her old boss in his new job or from working for a large charity as a consultant. The senior managers spent an average of £7,000 of their health authority's money each week on entertainment at restaurants and hotels. The report of the Public Accounts Committee into this health authority calls for 'those responsible . . .

to account for their actions'. It concludes that, 'We are deeply concerned at the catalogue of breaches of process, internal controls and national regulations. . . . There were failures of governance of the most serious kind which have resulted in the loss to public funds of millions of pounds which should have been spent on treating patients.' The managers are still out there touting for business, citing their extensive 'senior management experience and expertise' to attract yet other ambitious colleagues to mine this rich seam of health and welfare money (Butler 1997, Foster and Carberry 1997).

THE POLITICAL AND ECONOMIC ABUSES OF RESIDENTIAL CARE

We know that some members of parliament and other powerful figures do not consider themselves to be subject to the same rules and ethics as they seek to impose on others, so we must also understand that not all the policy- and decision-makers who are so influential in the area of health and social care, intend to follow their own guidance. They make policy for others. The welfare systems which they take part in setting up are not for them either; they are for others to implement and yet others to 'consume'. Some policy-makers have things other than the primary task on their minds – money, political and career advancement, status and power, and, most important, implementing broader, but covert, economic and political objectives.

The phenomenal growth of spending on private residential care during the 1980s, the transfer of responsibility for paying for that care to the local authorities (community care) during the 1990s, the closure of hospitals and the growth of private and voluntary health provision were all driven by the government's political and economic strategy (essentially no different from the strategy applied to the publicly owned mining industry and its work-force). Its long-term objectives were to destroy union power, to reduce the scope of public sector welfare, to generate private business opportunities based on an insecure, part-time, non-unionised work-force, and to sell off publicly owned assets. The health service and community care 'reforms' were major tools of government economic policy. 'Welfare' was, is and always will be a vast sector of the economy through which major political change can be achieved. 'Community care' has transformed employment in health and social care. Thousands of previously secure, pensionable, full-time public service jobs have been lost. They have been replaced by very poorly paid, part-time work which has few benefits attached, and by unpaid care given at home. Training for staff, standards in residential care, staffing levels and the transfer of local authority Homes to the private and voluntary sector are significant parts of an overall plan, the prime purpose of which had very little to do with promoting individuals' health and welfare. The government made 'transitional' arrangements to soften the impact of its policy and to disguise the underlying strategy. People (mostly women) in households without jobs were pleased to get any employment at any wage. Employers were free to exploit a desperate work-force and vulnerable customers. 'Policy' was then invented to 'regulate', 'train' and 'assure quality'. The policy élite of the social care sector were engaged in weaving a grand deception. Perhaps many of them were genuinely unaware of the parts they were playing in an overall plan, but most of them are intelligent enough to understand, with hindsight, that such ignorance was in fact, for them, a defence – a psychological defence. In defending themselves and the covert political strategy in this way, they betrayed the residents and staff who were to become the victims of 'care in the community'. Instead of implementing systems which would protect residents, they merely invented systems to avert criticisms of the policy.

TRAINING AND THE POLICY ÉLITE

The yawning gap between policy and practice, and between those concerned with each, exists in all areas of the élite club and its policy-producing organisations. The Central Council for Education and Training in Social Work (CCETSW) draws in to its committees a carefully balanced mixture of establishment figures and erstwhile radicals (who are qualifying for their membership of the establishment). The organisation produces an interminable stream of verbiage, stifling the open, creative, rebellious imagination of social work learning in an attempt to train a standardised, quality-assured, competence-tested workforce – and failing miserably and expensively. In order to survive, the colleges, universities and all social care training agencies have to agree with whatever is produced. National Vocational Qualifications (NVQs), the Diploma in Social Work and even post-qualifying training must conform to the CCETSW prescription. Huge, complex systems are laboriously constructed to carry these new qualifications forward. With each long-debated, meticulously crafted, confusingly 'clarified' change of words, of emphasis or procedure, hundreds of large envelopes pour out of the central offices stuffed with pages of updates which are to be added to the vast ring binders, telling you everything you didn't want to know about the qualifications. Each change sets off further activity as the news 'cascades' to all the advisers, the internal and external verifiers, the practice teachers, the tutors, the supervisors, the trainers, the managers, the assessors, the boards and committees, the training agencies, the placement managers, and – even – to the candidates. All the stacks of paper, all the meetings and conferences, all the launches and publicity, all the hard work and the employment of intelligent people . . . result in a trickle of dissatisfied, frustrated and unstimulated – but 'competent' – personnel. Students spend endless hours of anxiety and confusion trying to assemble the 'proof' of their competence in every conceivable area of practice. Many of the placements cannot provide the experience of practice necessary to prove competence, so much of it is simply fabricated to meet the requirements of assessment.

The council for 'education' in social work is no longer a force for change and development, for challenge and creativity; no longer an organisation which leads others to think and to learn, but another bureaucratic quagmire into which initiative and talent sink. Beliefs and principles – such as racial equality, awareness and justice – are by turns trumpeted, bureaucratised, imposed by procedure and dumped when the establishment finds the image unfashionable. CCETSW, with its passionless procedures and its smothering power (like a great wet blanket), has huge influence over every training agency and section, and through them over social care. Although most residential care workers have never heard of CCETSW, they have all felt its power. In residential Homes, much training and development which might take place does not because of the dead hand of CCETSW. Although the clear intention of NVQs in Care was to bring training into the workplace, and although in the few Homes which have wholeheartedly committed themselves to NVQs, staff are indeed participating in training and obtaining their qualifications, the unintentional overall result has been to undermine and reduce all the other training which was taking place in Homes. Training has itself become over-professionalised and specialised; to do it and to take part in 'recognised' modes of training, you must speak the language and 'standardise'. No one may assess, verify or supervise – no one may take any part in the production of this 'competent' workforce – unless they too have proved themselves to be competent. The hegemony of CCETSW's new model training is oppressive.

More and more training is concerned with certainties – with quantifiable, measurable, concrete actions, rather than with questions and dilemmas; but giving care is uncertain, and most of it is not measurable.

It is intellectually and emotionally engaging. It requires staff to think and feel, to wrestle with conflicting forces, to tolerate the anxiety of *not* knowing (Parkinson 1997). Residential social work is done 'with' people, not 'to' people. The search for certainty is a defence against the anxiety engendered by the inherent uncertainty of the work and the precarious lives of clients; it is also a defence against the angry, envious, reactionary attacks on the whole notion of the sort of social work which is practised in a mutual, enabling and developmental way. Things might be easier if social workers merely had competently to follow procedure to sort out problems, and if clients did as they were told as well. This is the logic of trying to do all the thinking at a level far removed from workers and clients and of issuing what amount to instructions. But if clients and their lives were so amenable to 'solutions', many of them wouldn't be clients in the first place and there would be no need for social workers.

THE CIVIL SERVICE ÉLITE

At the top of the social services hierarchy but below the level of government ministers is the Chief Inspector of Social Services at the Department of Health. An experienced and trusted ex-director of a local authority social services department is usually appointed to this senior civil service post. He or she has an extensive department or 'inspectorate', who work on policy and monitor the performance of social services departments. (The 'inspectorate' for Scotland comes under the Scottish Office.) The Social Services Inspectorate (SSI) is an arm of a government department and its central function is to oversee the implementation and monitoring of government policy. Although the SSI has the role of 'inspecting' all social service provision and the local authority inspection units, inspection in this sense is only part of its work. Detail of legislation is drafted by the inspectors; guidance to implementation is written by them, and they then advise on and monitor how the legislation and guidance are put into effect. Each year the chief inspector writes a report on social services, and many other 'end of term' reports are written on selected areas which have been inspected. The inspectors are usually skilful and highly intelligent people, and, like the chief inspector, most will have had direct experience of managing social services. Generally, their reports are well researched and thought-provoking, and some are very practical and influential (e.g. *Homes are for Living In*, Department of Health 1989). Their guidance is sensible and humane. Although the inspectors (men and women) tend to present themselves as distant and superior civil servants (they wear suits and carry briefcases), the small proportion of residential Homes which have experienced their visits have usually found them to be at ease with and genuinely interested in the residents and staff. Their comments are perceptive and helpful.

The inspectorate is the most powerful policy-making body and provides leadership in developing services and raising standards. However, all inspectors have risen to these exalted heights, and in doing so they have become cautious, conservative and unwilling to rock the boat. They deliberate before responding. They are reluctant to take a strong line and to *require* adherence to the standards they have promoted. They act as a buffer between dissenters and the government. They are bureaucrats par excellence. Placed where they are and knowing what they do, they also have the habitual guilt and fondness for secrecy of those who are implicated and feel totally constrained. Beliefs and opinions are kept well under wraps. They are reluctant to commit themselves to principles, preferring to deal in established policies and procedures. If someone from the level of a residential Home (a member of staff, resident or relative) contacts the SSI to draw attention to and get action on malpractice, he or she is are likely to get a brief, polite but cool response directing them to 'the proper channels'. You may hope that they will make enquiries about your concern and thereby attend to the problem, but you will not be told. They do not encourage such contact.

THE EXCLUSIVENESS OF CLUB MEMBERSHIP

There is little two-way communication between the Social Services Inspectorate and the living, working environments of residential Homes. The SSI gathers and collates information; it reports; it advises; it inspects; and it makes policy. It talks with others who are at the same level – not in the same club, but in the same federation of clubs. Wherever members of the other clubs are gathered together, there will usually be representatives from the SSI present. The directors of social services and of social work (in Scotland) have a club. The chief executives of voluntary organisations, of housing associations and of private care companies have formal and informal clubs. There are associations for social workers and social care workers, whose general secretaries are elevated to associate club membership. The local authority associations appoint representatives to become prominent and influential members of the policy élite. Favoured academics are members. Some of the chiefs of the campaigning charities are also admitted, but on strict conditions; most will be temporary members – included until they become tiresome and outspoken.

Generally, the business is done quietly and privately, though there are regular public events when the membership and its work are put on show. Conferences in prestigious venues are important meeting points. Clubs invite prominent members from other clubs to come and give 'keynote' speeches. Reports are launched and the press publicise the events. There are even 'gossip' columns in the social care press – who stayed up drinking all night; who played tennis with whom; who won the charity bike ride. To some extent members let their hair down and there is much amusement at the antics of 'delegates' in the febrile atmosphere of a residential conference. The informal conversations, the jokes and the real opinions of members are not for the ears of outsiders. (Members who attend are unlikely to be aware how revealing their behaviour is to those who live and work in residential care, and who know that when people live together – even temporarily – their chosen façade is likely to crumble or to become transparent.)

Of course, many members join the élite clubs (and it is hardly feasible to stay out of them once you have qualified for membership) on the honourable basis that they must participate in the development of the services which they manage or for which they make policy. These are of course valuable opportunities; simply staying away will not change any-thing and might well cut one's organisation off from important benefits. Occasionally, exciting differences emerge between clubs and even between members of the same club. There have been brief moments of public confrontation: for example, between directors of social services and a junior government minister who has been invited to address their conference, and between hard-up local authorities and some charities which are resisting taking on more statutory work from social services departments. However, these 'spats' tend to be short-lived and the public face of the policy élite is soon hastily made up again. If, occasionally, someone who is not a club member is invited to speak about an issue of the moment, and does so in strong and challenging terms, that person is listened to politely and apparently attentively, and often congratulated for 'raising such important issues'. (Beware the soothing compliments of those whose complacency you seek to challenge.) If the equilibrium of the conference is momentarily disturbed by such a contribution, calm and 'good sense' are soon restored by skilful management.

Much of the time and energy of the policy community is engaged in building façades. Repeatedly, politicians require them to produce 'answers'. Committees of enquiry and their reports are used first to soothe and dissipate public disquiet and then to masquerade as 'action', even though few steps are taken to implement the recommendations. During this process the politicians will be mouthing platitudes about 'ensuring that this never happens again' . . . and then it does. (For the last thirty years various aspects of residential care have been described with wearying regularity as the 'Cinderella service' following the uncovering of scandals. This Cinderella never even got to the ball! See Afterword, p. 246.) The policy élite who produce the recommendations grumble quietly to each other, assuaging their guilt by telling themselves that they must not get political, and that remaining in office is more effective than getting the push. Meanwhile, in residential care, what change does take place is led by people like Rachel (Chapter 4), who seizes every piece of legislation and guidance, and every enquiry report, finds all those parts which she can use to improve the service and dares anyone to stop her. Unfortunately, there are not many with her courage and drive; most residential care managers follow the example set for them by the timorous and ultimately self-serving majority of the policy élite.

Like any group of people working together, the policy community needs to become much more self-aware and self-critical. The apparent advantages of their jobs – comfort, status, high pay and power – lead to the constraints of isolation and a fear of rocking their boat. The director of social services who decides that she will spend as much time with her basic-grade (primary task) work-force as she does in élite 'club' meetings will find herself changing her views, her attitudes and actions, without having to make a great effort to change. She will of course become an awkward club member, but it is quite likely that she finds the overridingly male culture of club activities uncongenial in any case. (Although Janet was not yet eligible for membership of this club, her experience of participating in the life of two Homes was her means of changing, first, her own work and, later, the whole management of her division.)

If they intend to lead and make significant changes for the better in social services, the policy élite must consider radical and symbolic changes in the ways they themselves work. Would it be so hard to hold the next conference of directors in a recently vacated local authority residential Home, or in a school, or a camp? And would it be so ridiculous to send the next small group of care assistants who are going on a residential three-day training event to the five-star hotel the directors would otherwise have used for their conference?

There are good people with sound principles in the policy élite. They are not happy to be isolated and constrained by the rules and the social and professional conventions of their clubs. There are of course directors of social services who ask fundamental questions. There are inspectors in the SSI who retain an independence of mind. There are influential senior staff in CCETSW who are striving to extricate themselves and the organisation from the bureaucratic bog into which it has sunk. There are dissenting voices – even at the top.

We have seen throughout this book that in order to manage residential care with principle and dedication to the primary task, managers are likely to find themselves at odds with their organisations. We have observed how this struggle parallels the work of staff and the lives of residents. It is a struggle to 'live your life' as a client of social care services and it involves conflict with the people, events and circumstances through which you have become dependent. While we have frequently highlighted the positive and creative aspects of living in residential Homes, we have not ignored the reality of this struggle to survive and to 'live a life'. The policy élite must recognise that real change takes place only with the residents and staff in the Homes, and that all their efforts should be focused on the primary task of providing the resources and the legislative framework within which the struggles of residents can be fruitful and fulfilling. But it is very difficult to keep such basic principles in mind when your club does not admit residents or the staff who work with them; when you find you just do not have the time to spend in Homes; when you hear at your club conference the same recurring jokes about clients of your services as those you hear in your golf club; when you earn ten times what the skilful basic-grade residential worker earns, and you never have to think about the cost of food or clothes for your children. No matter what your previous experience has been, life at the top cuts you off from the realities of residential care. Unless you practise dissent, you will lose the capacity to make good policy and to oppose bad policy. Unless you spend time with residents and staff, and open yourself to the challenges they will put to you, your contribution can only eventually become élitist and self-centred. If you do not feel the contradictions and injustices inherent in your position – if your en-suite room at the plush conference hotel does not feel less comfortable as you remember the living conditions for residents in your department's Homes – your policy-making will inevitably further impoverish people's lives.

To make policy and to give guidance which will enable residents and staff in Homes to change residential care, you must update your own experience – constantly. This is done not only by spending time with the people who live and work in Homes, but also by a critical awareness of and sensitive reflection on your own life and work. Develop the very same thinking, feeling, professional and moral accountability which you expect of staff. Consider the discipline and commitment with which Hyacinth (Chapter 12, pp. 186–95) worked with Mr Scott. Expect no less of yourself.

Chapter 15

Inspection and independent outsiders: protecting residents

Little boy blue, come blow your horn . . .

Brenda's attempt to protect residents – What Brenda didn't know – Regulation – Inspection – The inherent problems of inspection units – How have inspection units performed? – The process of inspection – The other independent outsiders – Complaints procedures

Many people who have been abused in residential care testify that they had no one to turn to for help at the time. Neither they nor their relatives nor staff in the Home could make their plight known. If they tried to complain they were either ignored or disbelieved – and then punished or victimised for 'making trouble'. Although there are systems 'in place' to protect residents, again and again abuse has continued unchecked and concealed, until in some cases mounting evidence of malpractice and cruelty has eventually led to an official inquiry at which the victims have at last been heard.

It is against this background that we will now look at 'outsiders' of another sort – those whose independent position should in theory enable them to ensure that residents are not silenced by the institutional power of the care-providing organisations. The most important of these outsiders – the one given the power to take action – is the inspector, and we will consider how effective social services inspection units are in protecting residents from abuse. We will also consider how, when inspection is truly independent (and seen to be so), it can become both the support for and means by which all other outsiders could participate in the protection of residents and in the development of Homes. Later in the chapter, we will look at the other independent outsiders: the campaigning charities, small voluntary organisations, the press, individual independent outsiders, and the friends and relatives of residents. They can play a crucial part in preventing, investigating and exposing abuse, though their success is largely dependent on the efficacy of the inspectors – as we shall see only too clearly when reading Brenda's story with which we begin our examination of their key role.

BRENDA'S ATTEMPT TO PROTECT RESIDENTS

Noreen's younger sister, Brenda, who lived in a neighbouring local authority area, worked for six months as a part-time care assistant in a small voluntary Home for older people. Although she had never before been a residential care worker, she didn't find it difficult to get a job in this Home, ten minutes' walk from her own house. She asked about work there one day and she was told to come back the next to start. To begin with, she was paid in cash by the 'matron', and after a couple of weeks, when she was deemed satisfactory, she was put on the payroll. There were very few staff and nearly all of them had been recruited in the same way. Poor as the conditions and pay were, Brenda liked the residents and found a lot of the work very satisfying. Within days of starting, she could see that the way she chose to work was making quite a difference to residents' lives; at the same time she realised that the general standard of care was very poor. It was several weeks, though, before she began to understand that the care was worse than poor – it was abusive and cruel.

As a newcomer she was not at first 'initiated' into the regular abuse that was going on. She did not immediately understand that the screams she heard from the 'confused' residents were in fact screams of pain, because other staff told her not to worry and said that 'they' were always like that when they got up in the morning, or when they were taken to the toilet. Later she was shown what 'had to be done' with 'confused' residents. If they were dirty in the morning – and they usually were – they were first wiped with the wet sheets and then pulled from the bed, stripped of their night clothes and sat on the commode. The bedclothes were removed and the bed made up. The residents were then washed roughly and their first set of day clothes (from a common stock) were put on. Brenda was told that if you didn't force them you would never get them out of bed and dressed, and, since there were only two people working in the mornings with fourteen residents, most of whom were incontinent, you couldn't hang around. If the residents were to be got up and taken down to breakfast by 8 a.m. you had to 'pull them around a bit'.

Brenda also discovered that some of the screams coming from the toilets were caused by something even more horrific. The 'deputy matron' took it on herself to 'manually evacuate' residents who were constipated. This involved putting on rubber gloves (which were otherwise in very short supply) and inserting her fingers into the resident's anus to pull out impacted faeces.

The residents were short of food and were sometimes begging for drinks. After putting Brenda on the payroll, the 'matron' explained to her that, although staff were not well paid, the low pay could be compensated for by perks. These included taking the pick of the deliveries of food which a large, high-class supermarket sent to the Home each week with the intention and reasonable expectation that the relatively expensive items would provide welcome treats for the residents; but the smoked salmon, joints of meat, ice cream, cheese cake, fresh juices and exotic fruit and vegetables all went home with staff. The residents sometimes had the bread or the plain biscuits, if there were some left over after staff had taken what they wanted, but what the residents ate was not extra for them; it simply reduced the expenditure on essential provisions.

Residents who had no relatives visiting were completely at the mercy of the abusive regime. Brenda was increasingly disturbed by what she was seeing, and with each new revelation she became unhappier but more determined to stay. At first she just blamed the individual workers who did these things, but as she too found herself tempted to hurry the residents because time was so short, she understood how difficult it was to work in any other way. After a few weeks she spoke to the 'matron' about her concerns. She was told that the Home was no different from any other and that there was nothing to be done about it. 'In the old days', said the 'matron', 'none of these residents would have been in a Home, they would have all been in hospital. We just get sent the dross now. They're all incontinent and senile, and the committee haven't given us any more staff.'

Brenda was perplexed by many things – by the drunken doctor who visited weekly but hardly ever saw residents; by where the residents' money went to; by who was really in charge – but she became so anxious about the welfare of the residents that she came into the Home on her days off to check that they were all right. Other staff thought that she was odd and warned her against 'over-involvement'. Far from being the 'nice little part-time job' which Brenda had been looking for when she took it on, the work was becoming a more than full-time obsession, and while her family sympathised and tried to support her, they could see it was making her ill. She could talk about nothing else at home and was often in floods of tears.

Of course, the obvious person to talk with about her worries was Noreen, but though she loved her dearly, Brenda had wanted to do this job without the advice and instruction of her big sister. Noreen was the oldest in a family of six and Brenda the youngest. Fifteen years her senior, Noreen had been a bit like a mother to her when she was a child, and Brenda just knew that her sister would tell her exactly what to do.

On one of her days off, Brenda called at the Home early in the morning before going out to do some shopping for herself. She went straight upstairs to see a resident who was 'difficult' but of whom she was very fond. In spite of everything, the old woman still retained her spirit. She would fight and swear and shout, but sometimes she was quietly appreciative of Brenda's gentle care. As Brenda approached the resident's room, she heard her screaming and she heard the 'deputy matron' shouting, 'Don't you think you can scratch me, you filthy old bitch. I'll teach you a fucking lesson.' Brenda also heard a smacking sound. She burst into the room to see the worker standing over the naked resident beating her with her urine-soaked rolled-up nightdress. Brenda snatched the nightdress from the 'deputy matron', and, only just managing to restrain herself from attacking her, growled, 'How could you? Get out.' The woman left the room, protesting that the resident had attacked her and showing a long scratch on her arm.

Staying with the resident, Brenda rang the call bell repeatedly until the other member of staff on duty came to the room. She explained what she had seen and told her colleague that she was going to do something about the situation, and that the 'deputy matron' was not to come near the resident. 'If she so much as touches her again, I'll kill her.'

Not having a clue what to do, she rushed home and rang Noreen, who told her to write down everything she had witnessed that morning, then to ring the police, the chair of the committee, and the inspection unit and tell each of them exactly what had happened. Brenda had never heard of the inspection unit but it sounded to her as if this was exactly the sort of problem inspectors should be there to solve, and so she rang them first. She was put through to an inspector who said that it wasn't his Home but that what she had told him was indeed very serious and he would pass the information on to the right person who would ring Brenda at home as soon as possible. Next she rang the chair of the committee, who didn't sound at all surprised and said he thought things might have got a little bit out of hand. He was calm and unruffled, and he strongly advised Brenda against ringing the police because, he said, they would not understand and probably wouldn't be interested. He told her to meet him at the Home straight away.

Brenda returned to the Home. The committee chair had not arrived but she discovered that he had phoned immediately after he had spoken to Brenda to instruct the 'deputy matron' to go home, and he had asked the 'matron' to come in. Brenda spent an anxious hour waiting for him to arrive. When he and the 'matron' arrived at almost the same time, he told Brenda to meet with them both in the office. She began to feel as if it was she who was in the wrong. The chair said that he had already spoken with the inspector, who agreed with him that the 'deputy matron' had obviously momentarily lost her temper, but that 'it happens'. Because Brenda had chosen to 'make a mountain out of a molehill', the deputy would have to be suspended for the moment, 'until the fuss dies down'. He said that the inspection unit would not be investigating the incident and would be quite happy for him to do so, and to send them his report. Had she got anything more to say than she had already said on the phone?

Brenda was shocked. She felt completely alone and unaccountably ashamed of herself. Near to tears and panic, she remained silent. The 'matron' said that after all she was a new and inexperienced member of staff, and that unfortunate things do happen in the work, but that she would just have to get used to it. She mustn't take it on herself to contact anyone outside, particularly the inspection unit, without consulting the 'chairman' or her first. Fortunately, she said, he had been able to sort out the inspector before the whole thing got completely out of control. Frightened, angry but still silent, Brenda got up and walked straight out of the Home to her own home.

Even before she reached her own door ten minutes' walk away from the Home, she had already begun to doubt that she had really seen and heard what had been done to the resident. The more she went over it, the more she wondered if she had exaggerated it and if she had been altogether mistaken. There was no one at home and she rang Noreen again. When she heard her sister's voice she broke down and began to sob that she had made a fool of herself, and berated Noreen for giving her such bad advice. It had got her nowhere, she said. Gradually Noreen encouraged her to tell her what had been said at the meeting with the committee chair and the 'matron' . 'Did you write down what you saw this morning, as I told you to?' 'Yes.' 'Well, read it to me then.' Brenda read it and began to believe herself again.

Although Noreen had little faith in inspectors herself, she knew that in this sort of situation they *should* be able to investigate and take action. She advised Brenda to ring them again because, as she pointed out, the inspector for the Home had not yet heard Brenda's story for himself, and Noreen was inclined to doubt that an inspector would agree to the cover-up which the committee chair seemed to be proposing. She also told Brenda that she should still ring the police because what she had witnessed was a violent assault.

Brenda was trembling as she rang the inspection unit again and managed to get through to the right person. He sounded most understanding but he said that the chief inspector had discussed the situation with the committee chair and he had been told that there was no need to get involved at this stage. Brenda began to panic. She could not accept this. She demanded to see the inspector. 'I thought you were meant to protect residents. That woman will be back to work tomorrow and she'll do it again. You have got to do something.' The inspector agreed to see her, first saying he had no time until the next week, but then, at Brenda's insistence, he arranged to meet her late in the afternoon of the same day.

Brenda spent three hours with the inspector and the chief inspector. She tried to tell them everything – about the incident in the morning but also about all the other abuse as well. They took pages of notes and thanked her for having the courage to come to them.

With her heart in her mouth, Brenda went in to work the next day. The 'deputy matron' was not there. The other staff and the 'matron' were coldly hostile to Brenda; she felt as if she had been sent to Coventry. She got on with her work and took her breaks with the residents rather than with the staff.

The day after, she went in to work to find two inspectors doing a surprise inspection. The 'matron' called in another care assistant to boost the staffing and it was all smiles and second helpings throughout the time they were there. The chair of the committee happened to drop in midway through the morning and spent a long time with the inspectors in the office.

Brenda felt immense relief. At last something was being done. It seemed that the 'deputy matron' had been suspended and that a proper investigation was taking place. The inspectors took copious notes and wanted to look into every nook and cranny of the place.

Without the 'deputy matron' around Brenda was less anxious about the immediate safety of residents, but some things got worse because it became apparent that she had been the organising force behind the conduct of the Home, such as it was. Quite quickly, the vestiges of discipline, which had just about kept call bells answered and staff following some sort of procedure in their work, disappeared. Staff spent more time together in the staff room, office or kitchen talking and smoking, and Brenda, always keen to be with residents, became more isolated. She found she was doing nearly all the work when she was on duty, and even when she was just visiting, she felt she had to respond to residents who needed attention but weren't getting it from the staff on duty.

Having had high hopes of change for the better after the inspection, Brenda once more began to despair. After two weeks she rang the inspector to find out what was happening. He told her that they were writing the report and a draft would go to the 'matron' and committee chair within the next two weeks. Brenda was exasperated when the inspector explained that there would be a lengthy process of consultation and amendment to the draft report before a 'public' report was finalised and Brenda could see what the results of the inspection were.

Initially she had expected so much of the inspection but now she began to wonder if she should ever have said anything about the incident or the Home. The 'deputy matron' was not working at the Home any more but Brenda had seen her there a couple of times. The other staff continued to be hostile; even so, two of them had come to her privately and said that they thought she was right, but added hopelessly, 'What can you do?' Brenda had received several anonymous threatening phone calls at home and her new coat, hanging in the changing room at work, had been cut from top to bottom. She kept getting the feeling that it was all her fault, and that the more experienced staff were probably right – 'What can you do?'

Brenda hung on somehow until, four months after the incident, the inspection report was published. She wouldn't have known it was available if she hadn't been pestering the inspection unit to tell her. As it was, none of the staff in the Home got to see the report, and Brenda had to collect it from the unit.

It was fourteen pages long. Brenda found it difficult to understand but scoured it to find references to the incident. Although it was critical of many of the practices and procedures of the Home, and listed ten requirements and twenty-two recommendations at the end, there was no mention of what had happened. Most extraordinary of all, the final paragraphs of the report said that the Home 'continued to operate within the requirements of the *Registered Homes Act*'.

Noreen had been trying to keep in touch with Brenda throughout this period. Brenda was reluctant to talk and felt ashamed of how little she had achieved. She thought that Noreen would have handled it much better – she, Noreen, wouldn't have let them get away with it. Nagging at the back of her mind too was her failure to get in touch with the police.

Soon after she had read the inspection report, another care worker told Brenda that the 'deputy matron' was now working in a nearby Home. Brenda was seething with anger. As far as she could see, no changes were being made at the Home as a result of the report; care was even worse than when the 'deputy matron' had been there; and now she'd gone elsewhere to abuse more defenceless old people.

On the day the inspection report was published, the old woman who had been beaten was sent to hospital with pneumonia. Brenda went to visit her and sat holding her hand, crying and whispering over and over again, 'I'm sorry.' Three days after admission, the old woman died. When Brenda heard the news she handed in her notice and went home that evening and rang the police.

Again Brenda was interviewed for several hours and she signed a statement about what had happened more than four months before. The detective who interviewed her said that such cases were very difficult, especially since it was now so long after the event, and anyway the alleged victim had died. Even if she had still been alive, he added, she would probably have been unable to give evidence. Also it didn't look good that Brenda had given in her notice and that she was so critical of the Home. He said that it was unlikely he would be able to find sufficient evidence for a prosecution if the social services inspection unit had already investigated the matter. However, he would certainly look into it and let her know what the outcome was. As the detective was going, he began to ask Brenda questions about her family both in England and in Ireland. Brenda's husband worked for a motorway maintenance firm and they had three grown-up sons. The policeman wanted to know what they did and where they lived. 'Just a chat.' Brenda had been subjected to 'chats' like that before. As he left, she knew her allegation had no hope of proper investigation.

WHAT BRENDA DIDN'T KNOW

Brenda had no inkling of the power of the 'players' in this awful experience or of the connections between them – why should she have?

The chair of the committee was previously a prominent local politician who retained his contacts with and influence in the ruling party. As leader of the council he had fixed many deals and covered up many scams. The other members of the committee which ran the Homes were under his thumb and left him to make all the decisions. He employed his niece as the administrator of the charity in spite of the fact that she could barely add up, took three hours to type a letter, and was unable to take minutes at meetings. He was effectively in sole control of a £2 million business and awarded contracts to friends, bought and sold assets (Homes), and was free to organise the finances to suit himself. He had even set up schemes whereby small amounts of residents' personal allowances were taken in cash by his daughter.

The 'chairman' (as he was always known) had a direct line to the director of social services and to the leading members of the party in power. To him, the introduction of inspection had been no more than a nuisance since he could always 'fix' any inconvenient problems which arose. He was also a prominent member of his local Masonic lodge, so it was not surprising when his fellow member – the detective – readily accepted his explanation of the unfortunate incident involving the 'deputy matron'. They had also agreed that Brenda was a somewhat suspect witness.

Although he could not stop Brenda eventually telling her story to the inspection unit, on reflection he reckoned it was better that she had done or she might have been tempted to go to the press or some 'left-wing organisation of busybodies'. As soon as he had received Brenda's first call, he got on to the director of social services to make sure that the inspection unit didn't come sticking their noses in. The director immediately contacted the chief inspector to tell her to keep well out of it, and she in turn instructed the inspector to listen sympathetically but to do nothing until it had blown over. An unannounced inspection would certainly give the impression of taking appropriate action, but she knew that it would in fact delay any comment for several months. The 'chairman' readily agreed to 'letting the "deputy matron" go' and providing her with a good reference as the best way of preventing any further similar problems occurring in the Home.

The inspectors and chief inspector resented the way in which they were pushed around and their reports were censored, but they had allowed it to start in a small way when they were first established, and now they were so deeply implicated in cover-ups and collusions that they could see no way of reversing the position other than by leaving the unit altogether.

On receipt of the draft report, the 'chairman' had removed all direct and indirect references to the incident. He was quite happy to let the requirements and recommendations pass because he had seen most of them before anyway, and had no intention of doing anything about more than a very few.

REGULATION

This book is being written at a time when many systems of regulation – among them those to safeguard health, personal finances, and standards in public life – have been shown to be faulty. Warning signs about the safety of food were ignored for years in the (short-term) interests of the producers, big business and government; reports were suppressed, parliament and the public were misled, and the truth was covered up. In another government-inspired deception people were tricked into abandoning reliable pension schemes and putting their money into 'personal pensions,' many of which turned out to be very poor value. In both instances, fortunes were made by individuals and by 'respectable' organisations at the expense of people's health and wealth. Yet, when they 'opened up' the pensions 'market' the government of the day said that their principles were choice and better value, and they instituted systems which promised protection for the 'consumer'. While in each case staff were recruited to 'ensure' that the regulations were obeyed, it was an open secret within each industry that they were being bent, ignored and flouted. The systems of regulation and protection were put in place by some legislators (MPs) whose own probity was so much in doubt that they were forced to set up an inquiry into 'standards in public life'. Again, the dominance of self-interest and greed rather than 'public service' was long-standing, deeply rooted and widespread, and the suspicion remains strong that in investigating and judging themselves, MPs will offer up some sacrificial miscreants – the gross offenders – to appease public distrust, leaving the underlying causes of corruption intact.

In this context what hope is there for the 'consumers' of residential care? (The consumers are residents, prospective residents, and their families and friends.) We know, of course, that in order 'to ensure' the proper conduct of residential Homes, detailed regulations and guidance backed up by a comprehensive system of registration and inspection have been 'put in place'; but can they be relied on to protect residents? (We should always be wary when politicians and policy-makers use the phrase 'put in place'; it is intended to sound reassuringly solid and certain, but often boils down to a distracting flurry of words disguising the fact that in reality nothing has changed. See p. 98.)

INSPECTION

Local authority social services inspection units were instituted after a powerful combination of events pushed government into taking 'action'. (Note the parallels with all other legislation on consumer protection and safety.) In the 1980s a series of major scandals involving residential care and abuse of children led to nationally publicised enquiries into practice, and they in turn led to legislation – principally the 1984 *Registered Homes Act*, the 1989 *Children Act* and the 1990 *NHS and Community Care Act* (under which the inspection units were set up).

In some local authorities, inspection units have operated with admirable independence; in others they have not (Burton 1996). The original intention was to establish 'arm's length' units which, although reporting to the director of social services, would be independent of all the services and other sections of local departments. Only a minority of units were originally set up in this way and most of those have now been subsumed into the mainstream of the organisation. Local authorities seemed incapable of maintaining such independent sections within them and gradually nearly all inspection units lost their autonomy and thereby some of the authority required for effective inspection.

Inspection units were to be *independent*, to report *directly* to the director of social services, to be '*arm's length*', and to be '*even-handed*'. Even though important elements of the original guidance have been quietly ignored, some units have succeeded in retaining these qualities. They owe their continuing independence and honesty to their strength of leadership, clarity of role and task, and to the social services directors' determination to give authority to inspection. (There are parallels here, of course, with successful residential management.) Yet too many of the other units have succumbed to bureaucratic subservience. If inspectors fail to provide a supportive link and focus for independent outsiders (and isolated insiders), but instead become an obedient arm of a powerful organisation, they cannot do what they were designed to do.

THE INHERENT PROBLEMS OF INSPECTION UNITS

Many of the original inspectors and heads of units were recruited directly from the departments in which the units operated, and a large proportion were not residential work specialists by experience or training. As so often happens, 'field' (office-based) workers were seen to be more suited to this task, even though their knowledge was limited. They were prepared to learn the legislation and guidance, and to apply them. Of the residential workers who were appointed as inspectors, many were tired, disillusioned, or on the verge of redundancy from Homes which were closing and had not been found another job. Other inspectors came from outside social services altogether: people who had previously worked in administration, education or nursing. There was a lot of reorganisation going on in local government and there were people who needed to be found jobs; as a new 'growth' section, social services inspection was a relatively secure haven. The units had to be set up; many chief inspectors chose to take a relatively well-paid local authority job rather than be made redundant from their previous middle management post, and they were presented with a team of inspectors in much the same situation. Inspection units were often 'cobbled together' in this way. It is worth reflecting on what the unconscious motivation of directors might be for accepting such an uncommitted variety of personnel.

At the beginning of inspection, experienced registration officers were already in post. (Registration was established in 1984 by the *Registered Homes Act*.) They knew the legislation well but had not previously had the time or inclination to evaluate Homes in terms of quality of life (*Homes are for Living In*, Department of Health 1989) rather than the quantifiable basics of the regulations (although they did use *Home Life*, Avebury 1984, for assessing these basic standards). These registration officers then helped the newly appointed heads of inspection, many of whom were initially fairly ignorant of residential care in general, to draw up the new standards for each inspection unit. They leant very heavily on *Home Life* and *Homes are for Living In*, sometimes reproducing whole paragraphs and sections, word for word, in their own standards. Most of the heads of inspection and many of the other inspectors were learning (and inventing for themselves) a new area of local authority work. Having been ignorant and inexperienced, they found themselves in a position to 'create' social services inspection units and a new 'discipline' of inspection; but, in the main, they had never been professional residential workers or managers, and, with notable exceptions, even those who had been showed scant ambition and enthusiasm for the work which Homes were doing. Most inspectors came to the task with the attitudes and approaches which we have repeatedly identified as marring management throughout the stories told in this book. In spite of their fondness for plagiarism, the heads of inspection produced some excellent codes of practice to issue to 'persons in charge' so that they knew by what standards they would be judged. However good the codes were, the inherent drawback was that the inspectors themselves did not fully understand them. On paper – yes – they were generally well written and comprehensible, but in practice – no – most of the inspectors had little idea how they might be implemented. (Another example of 'putting something in place'.) So, many inspectors reverted to measuring rooms, checking records and counting staff. (Even in these areas they often failed to diagnose the underlying realities, and ended up being given and reporting the same information in a more acceptable format at the next inspection.)

Inspectors wasted no time in forming their own organisations – their own clubs (Chapter 14, pp. 217–19) – but this generally did not move inspection on. The meetings did not challenge orthodoxy; they established it. Inspectors soon became simply another group of social service professionals, protecting their jobs, guarding their car allowances and pensions, looking for promotion, and attending training courses and conferences which would update them on the latest SSI circular, EC directive, or health and safety guidance. Important as such technicalities are, they are secondary to protecting residents from abuse and promoting and stimulating exciting new ideas and practice. Where was the enthusiasm and commitment?

Chief inspectors became the 'quality assurance' experts in their departments. Some units are now inspecting day and domiciliary care, and a few have widened the scope of inspection even further to take in all social care provision, assessment and purchasing, whether run by local authority, or voluntary or private organisations. While such expansion is stimulating and informative for the whole unit, there is a danger that it casts a shadow over the inspection of Homes and the promotion of good practice (inspection's original task), and, yet again, demotes residential care – and even those who inspect it – to second-class status.

HOW HAVE INSPECTION UNITS PERFORMED?

There is no doubt that in some local authorities inspection has had a strong beneficial effect. Some councils have brought their own Homes up to 'registration standards', which, of course, they should have done in 1984 when they were charged with the responsibility to 'ensure' that all other Homes in their area met those standards. Many private Homes have benefited from the advice and support of inspectors, and see inspection as a helpful process. General improvements have been achieved in the more technical and procedural areas of room size, safety, hygiene and keeping proper records. Gross abuses of residents and staff have not been eliminated, but they have certainly been reduced in number.

At a time when corruption and self-interest are both suspected – and frequently shown – to have permeated public service, inspectors have had to work very hard for the level of trust which their job requires. However, in some departments, inspection units have become the toothless, blind and deaf lap-dogs of unscrupulous politicians and senior managers: toothless, because they will not enforce standards when told to 'ease off' by their bosses; blind, because they do not see what is plain for staff, residents and relatives to see; deaf, because they will not listen to complaints. The most common criticism of local authority inspectors is that they pick on the faults of the private Homes and require changes but ignore the same or worse faults in their own council Homes; in other words, that they are lenient with their employers' Homes and unfairly demanding with the competition. But if the employer, the local authority, is itself implacably opposed to council provision and has, as so many have, transferred its own Homes to private or voluntary management, the opposite bias may be being practised by inspectors under instructions from their employers. This results, for instance, in inspectors allowing themselves to turn a blind eye to understaffing, because their council has an agreement to buy cheap residential places for clients from a private provider who is now running the ex-council Homes. When challenged about staffing levels the private care company can claim that they are staffing to levels approved by the inspection unit. (Such inspection units are often seriously understaffed themselves.) Every inspection report is read and, if not approved, altered by a senior manager outside the inspection unit before it is sent to the Home for its approval and becomes an 'open' report. There is much room for manipulation and trickery, and, even when their attention is drawn to malpractice, the SSI, who should be monitoring the performance of inspection units, are unwilling to take action.

One of the worst aspects of inspection, as it is currently practised in some units, is the delay in reporting and following up urgent requirements and recommendations. Providers in all sectors find it annoying – even enraging – that they are not given the 'results' of an inspection sooner. They may receive the first draft of a report several months after the inspection visit was made. They then have a short period in which to respond before the amended report can be made public. In a good Home, it is likely that many of the things which were found to be amiss at the inspection are put right soon afterwards. Months later they receive a report which details these faults and requires or recommends the action they have already taken.

Not only are reports often late, but they use too much space telling readers what they already know. They describe the building and the area in great detail and sometimes read almost like the more flowery 'blurb' of estate agents: 'a period building which enjoys fine views over the park' or 'the tastefully decorated lounge has French windows opening on to an extensive, well-maintained, mature garden'. Many reports depend heavily on the information contained in 'pre-inspection questionnaires', simply listing figures and restating mundane data about the Home. Inspection is becoming routinised in many units. Inspectors are looking for more ways in which the visit and especially the report can become standardised. Whole chunks of reports and the letters accompanying them are already computer-generated. Computer software is available which takes the slog out of report-writing. Inspectors can write their reports simply by entering key words. Although it is sensible to save time retyping all the common headings and any common paragraphs (of which there should be very few), and although reports are more accessible and comparable if they follow a common format, the computer cannot do the thinking for inspectors; it cannot make judgements.

When you get to the body of the report – What is the place really like? What do residents and relatives say about it? What happens at breakfast time? Do residents manage their own money? Are there enough staff? – you may be disappointed by the lack of detail and real 'feel', and what there is can be quite obscure and couched in jargon.

When some inspectors come to write their requirements and recommendations they go to town, sometimes listing as many as forty actions which they are telling the person in charge she or he must do (requirements), or suggesting she or he should do (recommendations). These lists can get out of hand because if, as frequently occurs, five of the requirements and fifteen of the recommendations have not been carried out by the next inspection, logic dictates that some action is taken to enforce the inspector's report, or, at the very least, they must be added to the new list. Thus lists get longer and more impossible to accomplish.

Before making requirements and recommendations, inspectors should discuss their feasibility with all concerned and then make a judgement themselves. In most Homes, the inspector should consider the Home's stage of development and its capacity for change before deciding what are the absolute essentials (requirements) and what are the desirable changes (recommendations). The requirements will be confined to those things which definitely must be changed for the Home or an aspect of it to remain 'registerable', and the inspector will have thought about what action to take if a requirement is not complied with. There is little point in making numerous recommendations if you know that the Home cannot possibly achieve them, so it is wise and helpful to recommend changes which you have already discussed with the person in charge and have realistic hopes that the Home can manage. Good inspection is a dialogue about change.

THE PROCESS OF INSPECTION

Inspection should be a well-managed, open process, not a one-off event. It can – and quickly does – become institutionalised in the ways that some Homes are institutionalised. If inspection becomes too much of a routine – a chore for both sides to get through as soon as possible – it loses its creative potential for helping Homes to bring about change.

The process of inspection should be all-year-round: at times – during inspection visits and reporting – very much in the foreground of the life and work of the Home; at other times, a significant part of the background. Inspectors are required to make at least two inspection visits each year: one announced and one unannounced.

The whole programme of the announced inspection, if properly carried out, cannot take place over a period of less than about three months. The inspector should give at least one month's notice to the Home and agree a date for the visit. She should ensure that residents, relatives, visitors, community care managers, staff and anyone at all who has an interest in the Home know about the inspection and are able to contact her with their own observations and views. She will prepare herself for the inspection by reviewing previous reports and any information which has come to the unit since the last inspection, and by deciding on the particular focus she needs to take in this inspection. If the inspection unit has established itself as a familiar contact point, and the inspector herself is an easy person to speak with and is known to listen and to take comments seriously, then outsiders will be able and willing to participate in the inspection process. They make valuable contributions both during the period of the inspection itself and by contacting the inspector at other times of the year with their concerns – or, indeed, with their positive comments – all of which add to the overall, outside estimation of the Home.

By its nature the unannounced inspection will not involve the Home in the same way prior to the visit. However, the process following the visit should take a similar course and should include (in brief outline): writing the draft report and sending it to the Home for consultation; discussion with all interested parties including staff, residents and relatives; amending the report where necessary to incorporate feedback received on the draft and plans the Home has put forward for meeting any requirements and responding to any recommendations; and the publication of the composite, final report. When the report becomes public, there are likely to be further responses from outsiders who have not yet participated in the process, and there is continuing dialogue between the inspector and the Home as it makes use of the report in implementing changes. It follows that the two inspections, and their preparation and follow-up, will involve an inspector in regular contact of varying intensity with a Home throughout the year.

In some units, the introduction of 'lay assessors' (who are themselves meant to be independent outsiders), although strongly resisted by some inspectors, has been a boost to the independence of inspection. In units where lay assessors were experienced as an inconvenience, inspectors resisted having their inward-looking, professional cosiness disturbed and opened up. In those units lay assessors have made little impact. They are peripheral to the process. They rarely write their own reports but are asked to give their impressions to the inspector, who will incorporate them into the report if they agree with her own. In more progressive units, however, the lay assessors' contribution has been very fruitful. Of course, they need training and support (of a sort which maintains their independence), and the logistics of making mutually convenient arrangements are difficult; but lay assessors can bring a fresh eye and a useful ignorance which cut through some of the professional rivalries and collusions inherent in the relationship between the inspector and the Home.

Like good residential care but not nearly so complex, the practice of good inspection is achieved through clear management and administration. If an inspector is responsible for twenty Homes, all of which she must inspect at least twice each year, she will have to make an inspection visit and write a report during nearly every working week of her year. She will complete a minimum of forty inspections in the year. In addition she will join with her colleagues in planning the work of the unit; she will liaise with a large number of providers, managers, staff, relatives and residents; she will train and support lay assessors; she will go to innumerable meetings, including the regular meetings of the inspection advisory panel and meetings with staff, residents and relatives; she will write reports and summaries for the social services committee and she will attend their meetings; she will contribute to the annual report of the unit; she will keep herself up to date with the latest circulars from the Department of Health and with new writing and thinking about residential care and inspection. And while she is inspecting, reporting and taking part in the work of the whole unit, she will also find time and opportunity to attend to the needs of all those people outside the organisations with which she routinely deals. This area of work – responding to the anxious phone calls, the complaints, the letters of enquiry, the requests for help and information – is in some senses the inspector's most important contribution to protecting residents. It is the vital channel of communication which provides a link and gives a voice to those who are on their own.

People can get in touch only if the inspector makes herself available, responds promptly to phone calls and letters, and encourages the frightened neighbour or member of staff who won't give a name – and only if she has organised all the rest of her work well. A worried caller will get an inadequate response from an inspector who has four weeks in which to complete half her year's inspection programme. She will pretend to herself that she can do five inspections a week for four weeks, can write up her reports at night, and get it all finished in time. She hasn't got a hope of doing it, but in trying she will cut off communication with everyone (and most significantly with isolated, desperately worried individuals who are unlikely to try again). She will rush her inspections and her reports, and she will not retain the information from one day to the next because she will subject herself to a confusing overload of important observations. In fact, she will not have time to do anything properly. It will all be rushed and muddled, and she will spend the first two or three months of the next year completing the previous year's programme, so ensuring that she will not have sufficient time to do her job properly, even if she plans it much better.

We must question this inspector's fitness to make judgements about the management and administration of a residential Home. How could this inspector make useful and critical comments about staff deployment – rotas, annual leave, allocating time for attending to residents' special needs – when it is so obvious that she can't even manage her own work programme? We should also question the chief inspector's management of the unit. During the process of inspection, the way in which inspectors conduct and manage themselves determines the value of the inspection, and it also provides an influential model of management for the Homes. The quality of inspectors' contact with individual outsiders – their openness, accessibility and responsiveness – is the main determinant of their capacity to prevent or detect abuse.

Planning, managing and completing an inspection programme is a relatively straightforward job when compared with managing the primary task and the resources of even a small Home. Both the will and the competence to manage their own task are basic requirements of inspectors. Those who fall short of the requirements will fail to protect residents adequately.

To inspect well, inspectors need authority in the same way as good managers need authority (see Chapter 7, p. 70). Their authority will come from their principles, their knowledge, their experience, their independence and their honesty. It will also come from their professional and managerial practice – judged by other people's experience of the inspection unit in action. If there are doubts about these areas, inspectors will lose authority (or never gain it in the first place) and will inevitably resort to issuing ineffectual demands, orders and threats. While working *with* providers, they must demonstrate their independence *from* them. While working *within* social services departments, they must demonstrate their independence *outside* them also. Their professional self-assurance and authority will be enhanced by their capacity to be self-critical and open to criticism from others.

On first acquaintance, neither providers nor independent outsiders have any strong reasons to trust inspectors. The statements about their impartiality ring hollow until inspectors themselves demonstrate their single-minded dedication to high standards of care wherever it is being provided, and their willingness to help any Home at all to achieve high standards. Like cricket umpires, inspectors get reputations which are largely deserved. Their impartiality and authority are not established by becoming aloof or by being authoritarian. To do their job they must remain closely in touch with and on good terms with people, but it is they themselves who have to make a judgement. Sometimes they may just 'have a quiet word' about a tendency which they have noticed; later they may give a warning; only very reluctantly will they resort to disciplinary measures and lay down the law. They can and will make mistakes which are tolerable if they can admit that they are not infallible, and if the mistakes plainly have neither bias nor malicious or destructive intent.

Because inspection units and the structure of inspection are the statutory protectors of residents, all the other people and organisations concerned with preventing or detecting abuse are obliged to work through the units. It is very difficult to make progress without them; if they are not working effectively, residents are largely unprotected.

In recent years, there have been several examples of people or their families (e.g. the relatives of Stephen Lawrence, murdered in Greenwich in 1993) having to defend themselves or their communities (sometimes by pursuing private prosecutions) because the police or the director of public prosecutions failed to gather evidence or to proceed against criminals. If trust in the police to protect the public falters and a suspicion grows that some groups will be left without the protection of the law, it is very difficult to re-establish such trust. Very few individuals have the resources to do what the police should have done. It is the same with the inspection of Homes. Once a unit has shown itself to lack independence and authority, and is suspected of being under the influence of powerful interest groups, individual complainants have nowhere to go to. They have neither the legal powers nor the resources to investigate abuse (Burton 1997).

THE OTHER INDEPENDENT OUTSIDERS

The one hope for individuals in these circumstances is that they will find some organisation or journalist to pursue their case. Most people living in residential care and their relatives, friends and advocates are, almost by definition, people who are vulnerable and relatively powerless. One of the declared tasks of residential staff is to support residents in finding a voice and taking back their power (professionally called 'empowerment'). Yet we know this rarely happens; and when it does, some organisations providing residential care find it a problem. This is an inherent contradiction which does not need resolution so much as 'living with' – which is what happens in good residential Homes and, of course, in good families as children grow up – as family members' power and status change in relation to each other. In a poor Home the rights, voices and self-determination of residents are quashed.

Any manifestation of the latent power of residents is experienced by managers and the organisation as a threat to their own power, rather than as a sign of effective work and as something to be developed and supported. It is in such Homes that independent outsiders are most needed, yet most unlikely to be encouraged. In a good Home the power of residents is the life force of a fruitful therapeutic ecology, and it is likely that independent outsiders will be very much involved as friends, relatives, advocates, neighbours, inspectors, trainers and ... the man who comes to lay a carpet and asks if residents chose the colour.

As they have steadily closed their own residential Homes, several of the large child care charities have tried to establish themselves as advocates for the rights of children in care. In the 1970s 'progressive' local authorities were issuing charters of rights and contact numbers for residents of all ages, and yet continued to flout those rights and failed to listen to residents who were being abused. Large, powerful organisations have continued to 'sell' themselves and, of course, to attract donations and funding on the basis of their commitment to rights and empowerment. We have to suspect both the motives and the efficacy of such initiatives. Who are they for and what have they achieved? Unless the power of the organisation is challenged, and the committees and managers put themselves and their positions on the line, you can be sure that talk of 'empowerment' and 'advocacy' is mere window dressing. (Some of the work arising from such initiatives does sometimes challenge or at least embarrass organisations – a sure sign that it has been effective.)

The smaller campaigning organisations are open to the same charge. Often started by someone (or a small group of people) who has been on the receiving end of care, either as residents or as relatives, the initial motivation is clear. As they offer and get requests for help, the workload becomes impossible to deal with and they have to expand. They are desperate for funds in order to continue supporting their members. In the process of raising funds their original vision becomes blurred or distorted, often because the sources of funding are the very organisations against which they have to fight. The founders of the 'campaign' find themselves incorporated into the policy club (see Chapter 14, pp. 217–21); the number of paid staff expands; and quite quickly the organisation loses its cutting edge, becomes safe, and joins all the others which find their own survival more important than the original mission – they lose their independence.

Mere membership can have a dulling effect on relatives, who may join initially because here at last is a group of people who share the same

problems and concerns. After a little while they become habituated
to meetings, talks from professionals, and finding that they have a little
influence in the management of the Homes. All the fervour for change
and the demands that people's rights are honoured lose their attraction,
and members attend meetings for mutual support rather than militant
action. Such support is very important but it often means that the
upset and angry relative who wants to mobilise action for change gets
soothed and her anger is dissipated and lost. The wrong done to her
is explained away and nothing changes. The energies of such groups
frequently get channelled into raising money, organising outings and
arranging social functions. The members can become very closely
connected with staff and begin to think like staff – they become institutionalised and lose all pretence of being independent outsiders.

The charities in a position to retain most independence are those
which are sufficiently rich in endowments to provide their main income
and do not seek for ever to expand. They don't have to go cap in hand
to other organisations to survive and to do their work. Although they
may seek funding for special projects, they are not constantly looking
over their shoulders anxiously wondering if what they are doing
is approved of in the right places. However, their independence is
sustained – or compromised – by their managing committees and senior
staff. The danger is that people in these positions are already members
– or aspiring to be members – of the policy élite. Some of these charities
both provide truly independent advice and support to individuals and
lead campaigns for residents' rights and empowerment. However,
generally, they will not investigate and pursue individual instances of
abuse.

If, as so often happens, people find themselves trying to put right
a wrong and are looking for active, involved advice and support and
for help to change the circumstances of an individual or to expose the
malpractices of an organisation, they may, with much effort, be able to
get information but they are unlikely to get active help. 'Help lines'
seem to promise such assistance but in practice rarely offer much
beyond someone who will 'listen', providing useful information and
referring the caller to other organisations. This is what most 'help lines'
are designed to do, but when you are desperate for someone to 'take up
your case' and you do not know to whom to turn, something called a
'help line' sounds as if it might provide the sort of assistance you are
looking for. It doesn't! People in this position tend to get passed on from
one organisation to another – all of them wanting to help but unable to
do so.

The last ray of hope is the media. Contrary to popular opinion, it is difficult to interest journalists in residential care, and even if they do express interest, it is still more difficult to get them to investigate, and extremely difficult to get them to write or broadcast the story. Sometimes the campaigning charities can and do help. They cultivate contacts with sympathetic journalists and many have their own professional public relations officers.

With distinguished exceptions, journalists have the same prejudices about both Homes and residents as the general public. The abuse of residents usually becomes newsworthy only when it becomes public by means of an inquiry or criminal proceedings. There are very few journalists who will investigate and expose abuse, and who have the conviction and commitment to pursue wrongdoing in residential care. (Among the exceptions is Roger Dobson, who single-mindedly helped to publicise the abuse of children in care in North Wales and was instrumental both in bringing some of the perpetrators to justice and in ensuring that a full inquiry took place (e.g. Dobson 1997, Dobson and Sawyer 1997).

Media coverage of residential care is a risky area. In instances of abuse, organisations are quick to threaten to sue editors and many stories are aborted for fear of costly damages. Stories are usually based on proved and already published information which emerges long after residents have suffered years of neglect and cruelty. By the time the public reads the sensational news, Homes have been closed, and staff suspended or dismissed, and the managing organisations have prepared their defences and identified their scapegoats; it is far too late to protect residents from abuse.

If local journalists took the trouble to read the inspection reports on Homes and if inspection units were bold enough to publicise poor practice, there is a rich seam of newsworthy information which would both educate the public and would be highly influential in preventing abuse.

COMPLAINTS PROCEDURES

From the number of examples of abuse in residential care which do receive publicity and may subsequently result in prosecution and conviction (or, at least, may initiate thorough investigation but rarely effective corrective action – see p. 219), it may appear that a large proportion of the wrongs which are perpetrated by abusive individuals and organisations are in fact uncovered. The reality is that only a small proportion get beyond the stage where a complaint is registered, and they are themselves a tiny proportion of abusive incidents and situations which would be complained about if the structure of protection were more open and was designed to protect residents rather than organisations.

Inspection units were intended to be the principle means for preventing and detecting abuse. Apart from the visits they make to Homes, inspectors should expect to gather information from many other sources, the most important of which will be from individuals who have concerns. A major part of their role as protectors of residents will be performed by responding to, investigating and taking action on complaints. (Some inspection units do perform well in this crucial area; many do not.) The 1990 *NHS and Community Care Act* requires there to be 'complaints procedures'. However, many local authorities (and other large providers of social care) have constructed their procedures so it is now more difficult to make a complaint than it would have been if there had been no procedure. The common response to someone voicing a complaint is to present them with 'the complaints procedure', which includes filling in forms, timescales, letters of acknowledgement, complaints panels, appeals, etc. Such a procedure is daunting to most complainants, so when asked if they wish to make a formal complaint, they very soon back off. Organisations which operate like this are using the system to protect themselves. When a relative sees an instance of what appears to be poor practice and tells the manager of a Home, she doesn't want an inquiry or to get involved in filling in forms and giving evidence; she simply wants the practice to stop. If she feels she cannot go to the manager of the Home, to whom should she go? If she has heard of the inspection unit, she might well try them. What happens if they tell her that she must go to the manager of the Home in the first instance and that, in order to pursue her complaint, she must ask to be given the forms to fill in? What if they tell her that only when she has filled in the forms, and only if the complaint is not resolved to her satisfaction will the inspection unit become involved? It is unlikely that she will either make the complaint or make further contact with the inspection unit. This is not how complaints procedures are meant to work, but this is how many of them do work in practice.

Afterword: the future of residential care – an opportunity for change

There have been many occasions in the last thirty years when residential care has seemed to be on the brink of a breakthrough – when we could have converted the service into something to be universally proud of. Cinderella could not only have gone to the ball, she could have married the prince and lived happily ever afterwards. But it never happened – Cinders stayed poor, despised, worked off her feet and blamed for everything.

Practical demonstrations of the way ahead have been numerous. There are many important examples of progress: Homes like The Mulberry Bush (Dockar-Drysdale 1968 and 1973), Peper Harow (Rose 1990) and Inglewood (Burton 1988, 1989a and 1989b) are either still in existence or, in spite of being shut down, have had a lasting effect. Even now, progressive local authorities and other social care organisations are making commitments to high-quality residential care. (Lewisham Social Services have taken back the responsibility for providing good residential care for children and young people (Hume 1997).) We have some excellent expositions of principles and practice such as *A Better Home Life* (Avebury 1996), *Growing up in Groups* (Kahan 1994) and *A Positive Choice* (Wagner 1988). So what is needed to make the breakthrough on a national scale?

In this book we have analysed what is wrong and proposed how residential care could be managed well. In our stories several managers have succeeded in managing well in spite of all the constraints. It has been vital to focus on what has prevented good practice from becoming established in order to understand what it is that has to be changed; but in this afterword we will sketch out the way ahead without dwelling on the faults of the past and present.

REQUIREMENTS FOR THE GOOD MANAGEMENT OF RESIDENTIAL CARE

1 The primary task of each Home – to engage with and respond to clients' individual and group needs – must be clearly and concisely defined. The organisation and management of the Home must be individually designed to perform that task.

2 The organisation of which the Home is a part must give the manager the full authority and responsibility to manage all that goes on in the Home, all its resources, and all the transactions across its boundary. Managers must take on this assigned authority and must earn additional authority from residents and staff. Managers who try to impose their authority will lose it.

3 The manager must be honest in all ways.

4 The manager must engage directly – and support staff in engaging directly – with clients, and, as a team, they must respond to clients' needs.

5 Residents must be able to participate in the management of the Home.

6 Residents must be in control of their own money.

THE RESOURCES NEEDED

1 Staff must be adequate in numbers, and adequately trained, supervised and supported. They must be adequately paid and have good conditions of employment, and there must be a structure which is designed specifically to perform the primary task of the Home.

2 Buildings, furniture and equipment must be designed or adapted specifically to perform the primary task.

3 The Home must be adequately and effectively financed, and the control of the finance (the Home's budget) will be exercised within the Home.

4 All the practical aspects of the therapeutic social ecology – staff, buildings and equipment, and finance – must be brought together and managed within the Home as a coherent whole (designed to perform the primary task – to meet residents' needs).

THE FUNCTION OF OUTSIDERS

1 All outside management, administration and monitoring of the Home must be tested against the question: 'Is this necessary to perform the primary task of the Home?' Superfluous outside activity should cease.

2 The protection of residents from abuse should be the task of truly independent inspection units which are familiar and accessible to the Homes – to residents, relatives and staff. They will have the power to investigate and prevent abuse, and they too will concentrate all efforts on assisting the Home in performing its primary task.
3 All other outside bodies which are connected with residential care must serve the same overall function as the Homes do – responding to the needs of residents. They too must be judged on what difference they make to the lives and well-being of residents.
4 Finally, given adequate resources to do the job, each manager, each member of staff and each Home should stand or fall on the same test: 'Is this Home doing what it was designed to do and what it says it will do? Does it provide the service which residents need?'

Though they may not have been stated in precisely this way before, and though the emphasis on the manager's task within the Home may be stronger than before, these precepts are not new. To make a deep, lasting and widespread change in the management of residential care, the attitudes and practices of outsiders must change. In arrogating to themselves the responsibility for creating change in the service, outsiders take that responsibility from all but the most determined inside managers. While they may be able to create the conditions for change, they cannot, and never will be able to, implement the changes required.

The unpalatable truth – the principal barrier to change – is that there are superfluous managerial jobs to be lost and organisations to be dismantled. Some may be beyond reform. The development of residential care is stifled by the workings of outside organisations and the policy élite. Residential workers (including managers) must take the destiny of this essential social service into their own hands. Good residential Homes do this already. They know what their principles are and they are clear about their primary task. They then make policy and translate that policy into procedure only in order to practise – only to perform the primary task. The working-out of policy and procedure must stay within the Home, connecting principles, primary task and practice. If that work is removed from the Home, principles and practice are fatally disconnected.

Homes must set their own standards. Knowing their primary task, they will state what level of service they will provide; they will say how they will provide it, and then their practice can be judged on whether they meet their standards or not. Independent inspectors will ascertain whether the services meet both minimum national standards and the

Homes' own publicly declared standards. In addition, inspectors will help and advise Homes in developing their service. The process of inspection will be a plain and practical exercise, not an obscure and bureaucratic one.

The real costs of residential care – as it is now – must be calculated. The outlay is not merely the fees paid by purchasers to providers. The real costs include the vast expenses of ineffectual training (and of its damaging consequences); of community care management; of inspection and investigation; of state benefits for inadequately paid staff and their dependants; of the policy élite; of the health service provided to residents who are sick because of the inadequacy of their care; and above all the massive social cost of poor care – the damage to family and community life, and the direct damage to residents.

Having made a realistic estimation of these costs, we should compare that estimation with the full costs of providing an appropriate level of high-quality care for all residents. Employing properly paid, trained and supervised staff, with the time to meet the needs of residents, in buildings which are well equipped and maintained, with a fully responsible manager for each Home, will nearly double the fees charged for most residents. (The fees charged by children's Homes and some specialised Homes for adults are already about four or more times those for older people.) By reducing the hidden social costs of poor care, cutting all extraneous outside costs and charging the necessary outside support to Homes (e.g. inspection, staff training, etc.) directly to specified elements of the fees, the higher fees necessarily charged would represent the *whole* cost of the service and would be directly comparable between Homes and levels of care. In a very mixed economy of care, with all sorts of profit- and non-profit-making and public organisations providing the same service, the choice for consumers should be on the quality of the service within a small range of prices. Their 'choice' should not be made for them – as it is now – by community care managers who find the Home which provides the bare minimum of service for the least price – and by doing so drive quality down and charge the costs of poor care to other government and local government services, and to the family and community at large.

There is the opportunity to make these great changes now. With a change of government in 1997, there is the chance to change national social, moral and cultural attitudes to care. This opportunity is as much to do with entering a time of optimism and change as it is to do with some specific political philosophy. We do not want to go on reading about or seeing on television the iniquities of residential care; we should not go on being frightened by the prospect of us or our relations having to go into old people's Homes. *A Positive Choice* (Wagner 1988) must now become a reality.

Residential care (including nursing Home care) is a public social good, just as hospitals, doctors, clean air and water, cheap and efficient public transport, wholesome food, housing, education and recreation are social goods. These are resources which – directly or indirectly – we all need and use. Their quality determines the quality of life for all of us. They can be provided in many different ways by a variety of organisations. They must be well run, well provided – and well managed. Of course, residential care has to be paid for. We should not pay more than it costs to run the service properly (although private providers will take a realistic profit); but nor should we pay less. If we do, we will inevitably get a poor service.

If we do not take the opportunity now, we will miss it. In a short time we will sink back into apathy and depression – the Cinderella service. There will be more scandals and inquiries, more calls for change from the top, more policies and procedures – but still no action. The Marcias, Ellens, Noreens, Thomases, Rachels, Jeevas, Janets and Hyacinths will go on struggling – fighting to make it a better service. Within their own patches they will succeed – for a while; but if we take the opportunity, they will lead a change that will transform, enrich and elevate our whole society.

Bibliography

This bibliography contains the books and articles which are referred to in the text and many others which are known to have influenced the author while writing this book. It is not a comprehensive bibliography of residential care.

Adams, R. (1996) *Social Work and Empowerment*, Basingstoke: Macmillan.
Ahmed, B. (1990) *Black Perspectives in Social Work*, Birmingham: Venture Press.
Allen, I. (ed.) (1990) *Inspection Units and Complaints Procedures*, London: Policy Studies Institute.
Argyris, C. (1994) 'Good communication that blocks learning', *Harvard Business Review*, July–August 1994.
Atherton, J. (1986) *Professional Supervision in Group Care*, London: Tavistock.
—— (1989) *Interpreting Residential Life*, London: Tavistock/Routledge.
Avebury, K. (chair) (1984) *Home Life*, London: Centre for Policy on Ageing.
—— (chair) (1996) *A Better Home Life*, London: Centre for Policy on Ageing.
Axline, V. (1972) *Dibs: in Search of Self*, Harmondsworth: Penguin.
British Association of Social Workers (BASW) (1978) *Residential Care, Staffing and Training*, Social Services Liaison Group working party report, Birmingham: BASW.
Beedell, C. (1970) *Residential Life with Children*, London: Routledge & Kegan Paul.
—— (1993) *Poor Starts, Lost Opportunities, Hopeful Outcomes*, London: Charterhouse Group.
Bennis, W. (1994) *An Invented Life*, London: Century.
Benson, J. (1987) *Working More Creatively with Groups*, London: Tavistock.
Berry, J. (1975) *Daily Experiences in Residential Life*, London: Routledge & Kegan Paul.
Bion, W. (1968, 1980) *Experiences in Groups*, London: Tavistock.
Birbalsingh, F. (ed.) (1996) *Frontiers of Caribbean Literature in English*, London: Macmillan.
Bornat, J., Pereira, C., Pilgrim, D. and Williams, F. (eds) (1993) *Community Care: A Reader*, London: Macmillan.
Bowlby, J. (1971) *Attachment*, Harmondsworth: Pelican.

—— (1979) *The Making and Breaking of Affectional Bonds*, London: Tavistock.

Brearley, C. (1990) *Working in Residential Homes for Elderly People*, London: Tavistock/Routledge.

Bright, L. (1995) *Care Betrayed*, London: Counsel & Care.

Brook, E. and Davis, A. (eds) (1985) *Women, the Family and Social Work*, London: Tavistock.

Brown, A. and Clough, R. (eds) (1989) *Groups and Groupings*, London: Tavistock/Routledge.

Burgess, H. (1992) *Problem-led Learning in Social Work*, London: Whiting & Birch.

Burn, M. (1956) *Mr Lyward's Answer*, London: Hamish Hamilton.

Burton, J. (1988) 'Residential care: change from the inside' (a series of five articles), *Social Work Today*, 28 January–10 March.

—— (1989a) 'Making it work: group living in residential care' (a series of four articles), *Social Work Today*, 6 April–18 May.

—— (1989b) 'Institutional change and group action: the significance and influence of groups in developing new residential services for older people', in A. Brown and R. Clough (eds) *Groups and Groupings*, London: Tavistock/ Routledge.

—— (1990) 'Speaking for ourselves', 'Rule from the inside out', 'Plugging into user power' (a series of three articles), *Care Weekly*, 13–27 July.

—— (1993) *The Handbook of Residential Care*, London: Routledge.

—— (1996) 'Out of the dark', *Community Care*, 7–13 March.

—— (1997) 'Listen to relatives on Wandsworth staff cuts' (letter), *Community Care*, 6–12 March.

Busby, M. (ed.) (1992) *Daughters of Africa*, London: Vintage.

Butler, P. (1997) '"Yorkshiregate" report attacks former RHA chair', *Health Service Journal*, 27 March.

Carter, N., Klein, R. and Day, P. (1992) *How Organisations Measure Success*, London: Routledge.

Castle Priory Study Group (1969) *The Residential Task in Child Care*, London: Residential Child Care Association.

Central Council for Education and Training in Social Work (CCETSW) (1973) *Training for Residential Work*, London: CCETSW.

—— (1973) *Residential Work is a Part of Social Work*, London: CCETSW.

Clark, N. (1991) *Managing Personal Learning and Change*, London: McGraw-Hill.

Clough, R. (1981) *Old Age Homes*, London: George Allen & Unwin.

—— (1982) *Residential Work*, Basingstoke: Macmillan.

—— (ed.) (1994) *Insights into Inspection*, London: Whiting & Birch/Social Care Association (Education).

Clutterbuck, D. and Dearlove, D. (1996) *The Charity as a Business*, London: Directory of Social Change.

Cockburn, C. (1977) *The Local State*, London: Pluto.

Cohen, S. (1985) *Visions of Social Control*, Cambridge: Polity.

Coulshed, V. (1990) *Management in Social Work*, Basingstoke: Macmillan.

Counsel & Care (1991) *Not Such Private Places*, London: Counsel & Care.

—— (1992) *What if they Hurt themselves?*, London: Counsel & Care.

—— (1993) *The Right to Take Risks*, London: Counsel & Care.

Craib, I. (1994) *The Importance of Disappointment*, London: Routledge.

Curle, A. (1990) *Tools for Transformation*, Stroud: Hawthorn Press.

Dartington, T., Miller, E. and Gwynne, G. (1981) *A Life Together*, London: Tavistock.

Davis, L. (1982) *Residential Care: a Community Resource*, London: Heinemann.

Dearling, A. (1991) *Effective Use of Teambuilding*, Harlow: Longman.

De Board, R. (1978) *The Psychoanalysis of Organisations*, London: Tavistock.

Department of Health (1989) *Caring for People: Community Care in the Next Decade and Beyond*, London: HMSO.

—— (1989) *Homes are for Living In*, London: HMSO.

—— (1991) *The Children Act 1989: Guidance and Regulations: vol. 4, Residential Care*, London: HMSO.

—— (1991) *Children in the Public Care*, London: HMSO.

Dharamsi, F., Edmonds, G., Filkin, E., Headley, C., Jones, P., Naish, M., Scott, I., Smith, E., Smith, H. and Williams, J. (1979) *Community Work and Caring for Children*, Ilkley: Owen Wells.

Dobson, R. (1997) 'Eighty names as child abusers in Clwyd inquiry', *The Independent on Sunday*, 19 January.

Dobson, R. and Sawyer, P. (1997) 'Clwyd: at long last the cover-up is over', *The Independent on Sunday*, 19 January.

Dockar-Drysdale, B. (1968) *Therapy in Child Care*, London: Longman.

—— (1973) *Consultation in Child Care*, London: Longman.

Douglas, R. and Payne, C. (1987) *Learning about Caring* (four sections), London: National Institute for Social Work (NISW).

—— (1988) *Organising for Learning*, London: National Institute for Social Work (NISW).

Douglas, T. (1986) *Group Living*, London: Tavistock.

—— (1995) *Scapegoats*, London: Routledge.

Drucker, P. (1979) *Management*, London: Pan.

Ford, K. and Hargreaves, S. (1991) *First Line Management: Staff*, Harlow: Longman.

Foster, J. and Carberry, J. (1997) 'Health body excesses appal MPs', *Evening Press* (York), 26 March.

Fox, E.M. and Urwick, L. (eds) (1973) *Dynamic Administration: the Collected Papers of Mary Parker Follett*, London: Pitman.

Francis, D. (1990) *Effective Problem-Solving*, London: Tavistock.

Fryer, P. (1984) *Staying Power: the History of Black People in Britain*, London: Pluto.

Gibson, T. (1996) *The Power in Our Hands*, Charlbury: Jon Carpenter.

Gilroy, B. (1986) *Frangipani House*, London: Heinemann.

Gilroy, P. (1987) *There Ain't No Black in the Union Jack*, London: Hutchinson.

Goffman, E. (1961, 1968) *Asylums*, Harmondsworth: Pelican.

Goward, L. (1995) *At the Public's Convenience*, London: Counsel & Care.

Graham, P. (1991) *Integrative Management*, Oxford: Blackwell.

Griffiths, R. (1988) *Community Care: Agenda for Action*, London: HMSO.

Grimwood, C. and Popplestone, R. (1993) *Women, Management and Care*, London: Macmillan.

Handy, C. (1990) *Inside Organizations*, London: BBC.

Harris, J. and Kelly, D. (1991) *Management Skills in Social Care*, Aldershot: Gower.

Hawkins, P. (1989) 'The social learning approach to residential and day care', in A. Brown and R. Clough (eds) *Groups and Groupings*, London: Tavistock/ Routledge.

Hawkins, P. and Shohet, R. (1989) *Supervision in the Helping Professions*, Buckingham: Open University.

Hayes, J. (1996) *Developing the Manager as Helper*, London: Routledge.

Heath, R. (1991) *Shadows Round the Moon*, London: Fontana.

Herman, S. and Korenich, M. (1977) *Authentic Management*, London: Addison-Wesley.

Hill, S. (1990) *More than Rice and Peas*, London: Food Commission.

hooks, b. (1995) *Killing Rage – Ending Racism*, London: Penguin.

Hope, P. (1992) *Making the Best Use of Consultants*, Harlow: Longman.

Hume, C. (1997) 'Good homes of our own', *Guardian*, 8 January.

Humphreys, M. (1994) *Empty Cradles*, London: Doubleday.

Illich, I. (1973) *Celebration of Awareness*, Harmondsworth: Penguin.

Itzin, C. and Newman, J. (1995) *Gender, Culture and Organizational Change*, London: Routledge.

Jenkins, D. (1996) *Managing Empowerment*, London: Century.

Jones, H. (1978) *The Residential Community: a Setting for Social Work*, London: Routledge & Kegan Paul.

Jones, M. (1979) 'The therapeutic community, social learning and social change', in R.D. Hinshelwood and N. Manning (eds) *Therapeutic Communities*, London: Routledge & Kegan Paul.

Jordan, J. (1987) *Moving Towards Home: Political Essays*, London: Virago.

Kahan, B. (1994) *Growing up in Groups*, London: HMSO.

Knapp, M. (1984) *The Economics of Social Care*, London: Macmillan.

Landau, M. and Stout, R. (1979) 'To manage is not to control: or the folly of Type II Errors', *Public Administration Review*, March/April.

Landry, C., Morley, D., Southwood, R. and Wright, P. (1985) *What a Way to Run a Railroad*, London: Comedia.

Lane, D. (1980) *Staffing Ratios in Residential Establishments*, London: Residential Care Association.

Levi, P. (1987) *Moments of Reprieve*, London: Sphere.

Marris, P. (1986) *Loss and Change*, London: Routledge & Kegan Paul.

Martin, S. (1983) *Managing without Managers*, London: Sage.

Menzies, I. (1970) *The Functioning of Social Systems as a Defence Against Anxiety*, Tavistock pamphlet no. 3, London: Tavistock.

Menzies Lyth, I. (1988) *Containing Anxiety in Institutions*, London: Free Association Books.

—— (1989) *The Dynamics of the Social*, London: Free Association Books.

Morgan, G. (1986) *Images of Organization*, London: Sage.

—— (1989) *Creative Organization Theory*, London: Sage.

Mulgen, G. (1988) 'The power of the weak', *Marxism Today*, December.

Newton, N. (1980) *This Bed my Centre*, London: Virago.

Obholzer, A. and Roberts, V.Z. (eds) (1994) *The Unconscious at Work*, London: Routledge.

Oni, O. (1997) *Who Should Run the Health Service?*, Oxford: Radcliffe.

Parkinson, C. (1997) *Competence in Social Work Education: but how are we learning?* Monograph series, London: University of East London.

Pedlar, M., Burgoyne, J. and Boydell, T. (1986) *A Manager's Guide to Self-Development*, London: McGraw-Hill.

Pedlar, M. (1996) *Action Learning for Managers*, London: Lemos & Crane.

Peters, T. (1989) *Thriving on Chaos*, London: Pan.

—— (1992) *Liberation Management*, London: Macmillan.

—— (1994) *The Tom Peters Seminar*, London: Macmillan.

Phillipson, C. and Walker, A. (eds) (1986) *Ageing and Social Policy*, Aldershot: Gower.

Preston-Shoot, M. and Agass, D. (1990) *Making Sense of Social Work*, Basingstoke: Macmillan.

Reason, P. (1984) 'Is organization development possible in power cultures?' in A. Kakabadse and C. Parker (eds) *Power, Politics and Organizations: A Behaviour Science View*, Chichester: Wiley.

Redl, F. (1966) *When we Deal with Children*, New York: Free Press.

Redl, F. and Wineman, D. (1965) *Controls from Within*, New York: Free Press.

Residential Forum (1996) *Creating a Home from Home*, London: Residential Forum.

Richards, B. (ed.) (1989) *Crises of the Self*, London: Free Association Books.

Rose, M. (1990) *Healing Hurt Minds*, London: Routledge.

Salzberger-Wittenberg, I. (1970) *Psycho-Analytical Insights and Relationships: A Kleinian Approach*, London: Routledge & Kegan Paul.

Schein, E. (1988) *Process Consultation*, Wokingham: Addison Wesley.

Segal, J. (1985) *Phantasy in Everyday Life*, Harmondsworth: Penguin.

Semler, R. (1993) *Maverick*, London: Century.

Senior, B. (1989) 'Residential care: what hope for the future?' in M. Langan and P. Lee (eds) *Radical Social Work Today*, London: Unwin.

Skinner, A. (1992) *Another Kind of Home: A Review of Residential Child Care*, Edinburgh: HMSO.

Sparks, I. (1997) 'Private providers versus local authorities', *Guardian*, 29 January.

Stewart, R. (1972) *The Reality of Organizations*, London: Pan.

Terkel, S. (1993) *Race*, London: Minerva.

Ungerson, C. (1987) *Policy is Personal*, London: Tavistock.

Wagner, G. (chair) (1988) *A Positive Choice*, London: National Institute for Social Work (NISW) HMSO.

Wagner Development Group (1990) *Staffing in Residential Care Homes*, London: National Institute for Social Work.

Ward, A. (1993) 'The large group: the heart of the system in group care', *Groupwork*, 6 (1).

—— (1993) *Working in Group Care*, Birmingham: Venture.

—— (1995) 'The "Matching Principle": exploring connections between practice and training in therapeutic child care', *Journal of Social Work Practice*, 9 (1 and 2).

Ward, C. (1982) *Anarchy in Action*, London: Freedom.

Warner, N. (1992) *Choosing with Care*, London: HMSO.

Wheatley, M. (1994) *Leadership and the New Science*, San Francisco: Berrett-Koehler.

Widgery, D. (1989) *Preserving Disorder*, London: Pluto.

Williams, A. (1991) *Forbidden Agendas: Strategic Action in Groups*, London: Routledge.

Wills, D. (1971) *Spare the Child*, Harmondsworth: Penguin.

Winnicott, C. (1971) *Child Care and Social Work*, London: Bookstall Services.

Winnicott, D. (1964) *The Child, the Family and the Outside World*, Harmondsworth: Penguin.

—— (1978) *The Family and Individual Development*, London: Tavistock.

Worsley, J. (1989) *Taking Good Care*, London: Age Concern.

—— (1992) *Good Care Management*, London: Age Concern.

Index

The reader is strongly advised to use the contents pages (pp. v–viii) to identify and locate the principal and subsiduary subject areas of this book. This index is designed to direct you to specific references within those broader areas but it does not list all the subjects in the contents. You will also find that there are frequent cross-references within the text to direct you to other parts of the book where the issue you are reading about is illustrated by an example or discussed under a different heading.